AF584827

IN THIS BODY

A BOOK ABOUT SELF-LOVE AND ACCEPTANCE

BY RUBY JONES

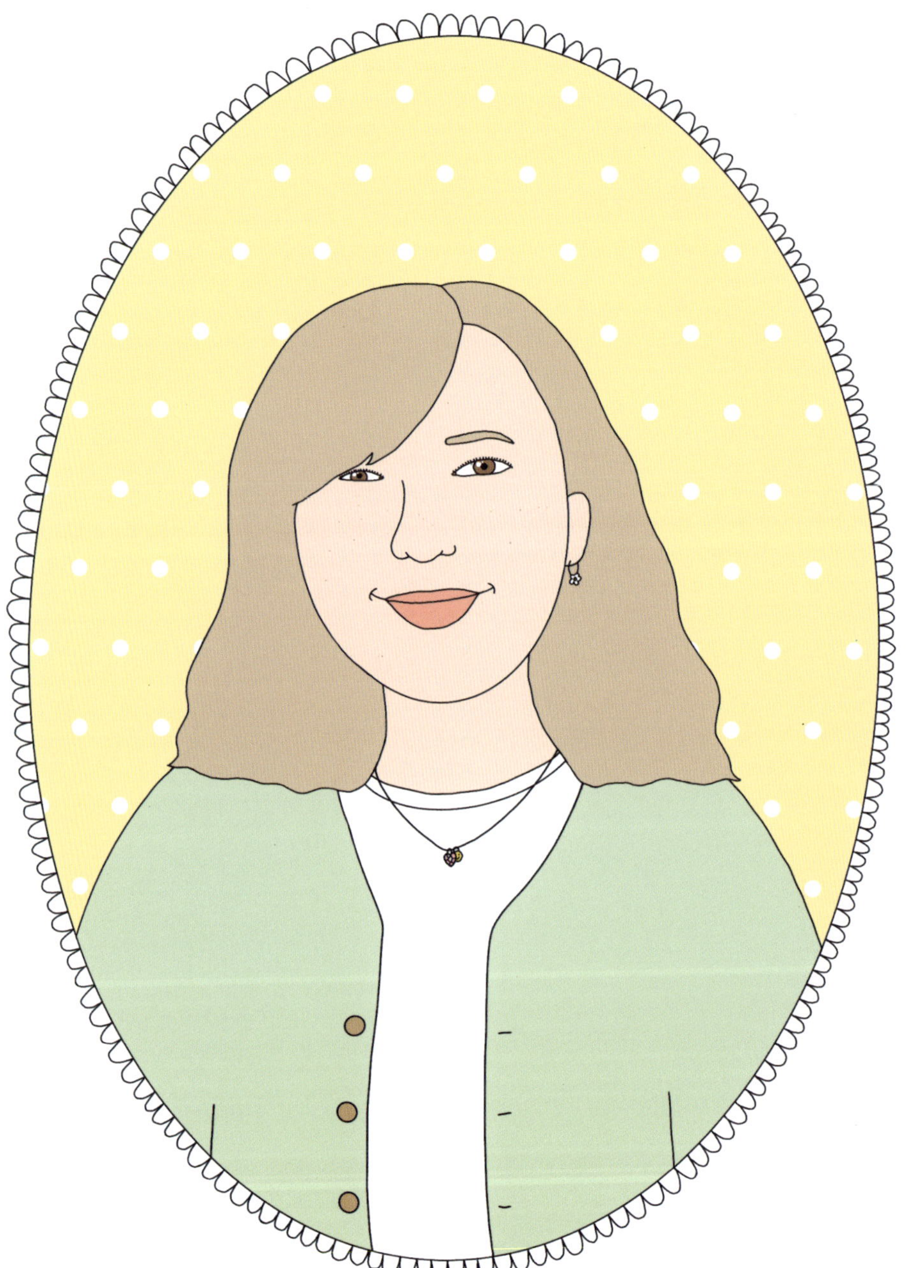

INTRODUCTION

When I was born I was sent home from the hospital just like every other healthy baby. It wasn't until they had me home, all to themselves away from the busy day in the maternity ward, that my parents noticed something. My eyes just seemed — different. Quiet enquiries ramped up to urgent responses from consultants who knew what it meant, and I had my first surgery at three weeks old. There were complications and more surgeries in my first year and then on into childhood, all in an attempt to preserve as much of my vision as possible. The end result was almost no vision in one eye and pretty poor out of the other, but I have made it work.

When I was really young, I didn't feel any different to other kids and I seemed to be able to do most things while wearing my glasses or contacts. Without them, unfamiliar places were scary and I would slide my feet trying to feel where the surface changed or find the steps before they tricked me. As I got older, I began to realise not only did I see the world differently to everyone else but I looked a little different to everyone else too. My eyes were uneven, murky and full of scars. My glasses were huge and thick. I was oblivious to the bigger picture — how lucky I was to have the vision I had, how lucky I was to live in a country that allowed me free healthcare, how lucky I was to have a family that loved me and only ever believed in me.

Heading into my teenage years, the way I saw myself spiralled downwards and before long I thought everything was wrong with me — my legs were too thick, my arms were too hairy, my smile was too gummy, my hips were too wide. I could find something wrong with every single part of me. This warped view of myself soon led to a quiet eating disorder and years of obsession around my body. While I have recovered and reached a place of forgiveness within myself, I know the relationship with my body is still a work in progress.

While the body positivity and self-love movements of recent times have filled me with joy, there are times when I find myself wondering where people like me fit into it all. Because I'm quiet. Because I'm shy. Because my confidence doesn't fill the room. Because, in all honesty, the love I feel for myself isn't always big and gooey and warm and endless. Some days it's tiny. Some days, I have to work really hard to find any at all. While I have more love for myself now than ever, it doesn't mean that some days aren't hard. That's the reality of being in a body that grows, changes and ages — like everyone else's — but with its own story, with its own hiccups and blemishes.

No one knows what it's like to be in your body, and no one has the right to tell you how to feel, act or exist in that body. You're on your own journey. It's your choice to share it or guard it closely, to be still with it or noisy, to laugh or cry at it — maybe sometimes both. Whatever you do, please take the time to marvel at it, to celebrate it, to love it. Take all the time you need.

Ruby Jones

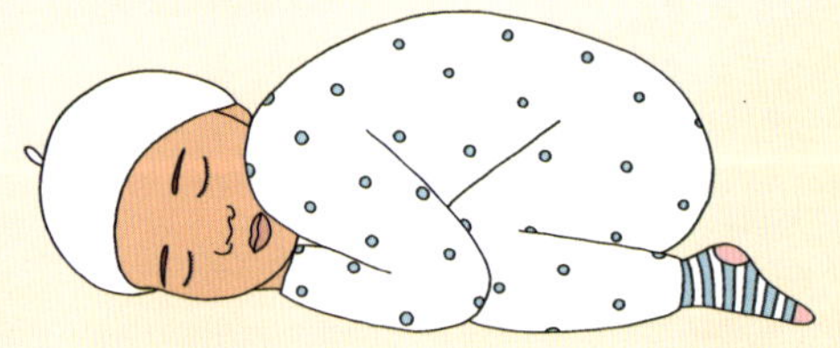

WHEN WE ENTER THIS WORLD,

WE DON'T HAVE A SAY IN THE BODY

WE'RE BORN INTO.

WE JUST DO OUR BEST

WITH WHAT WE HAVE.

AS WE GROW, WE FEEL THE EXCITEMENT OF BEING IN A BODY AND SPEND EACH DAY LEARNING WHAT OUR BODY CAN DO FOR US.

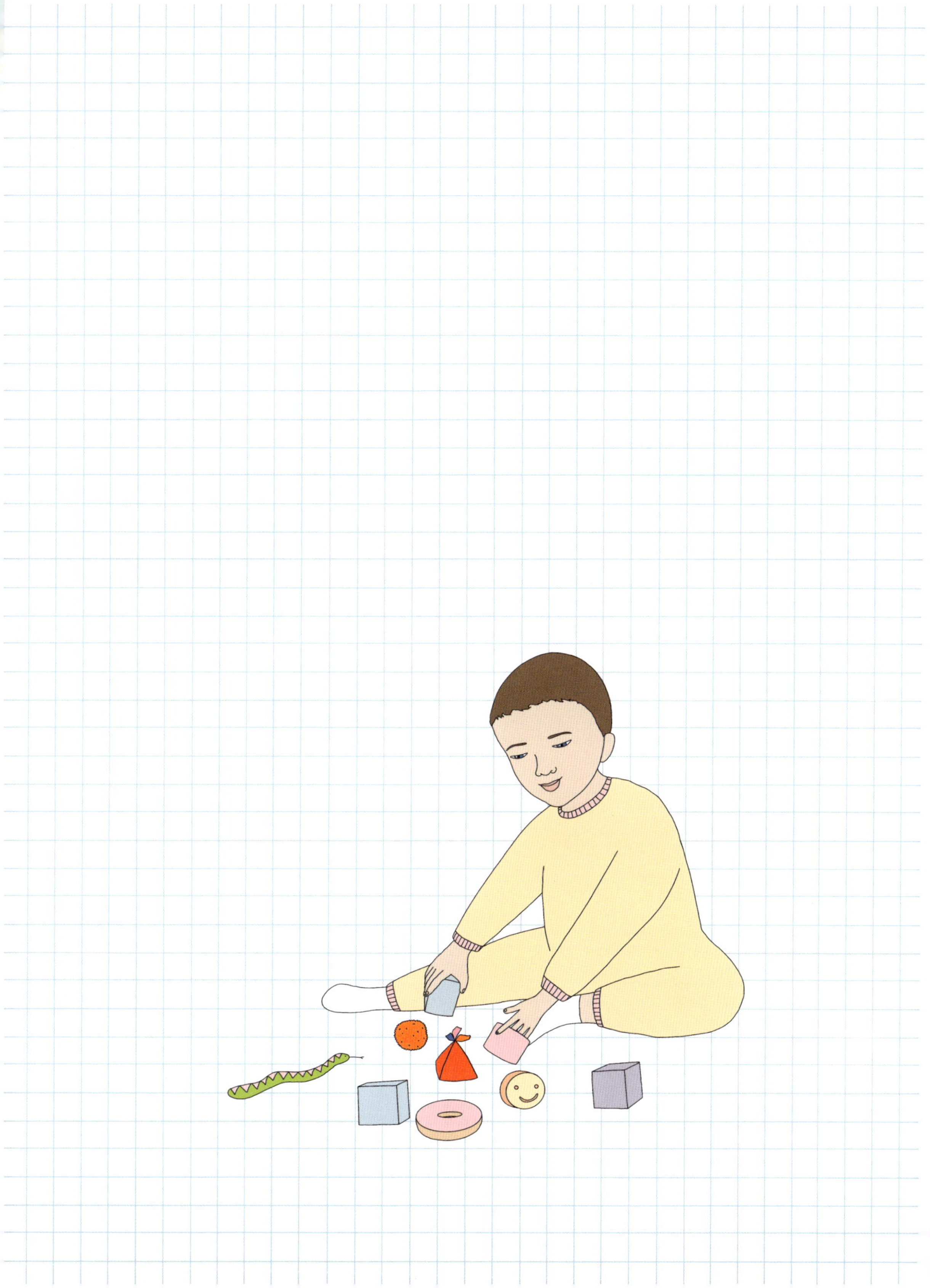

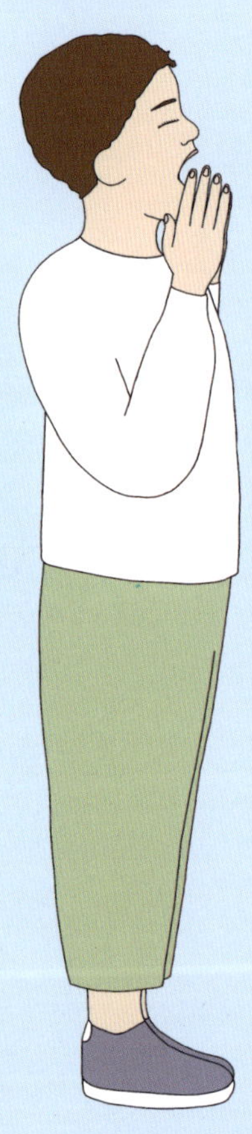
WE LEARN TO USE OUR VOICE...

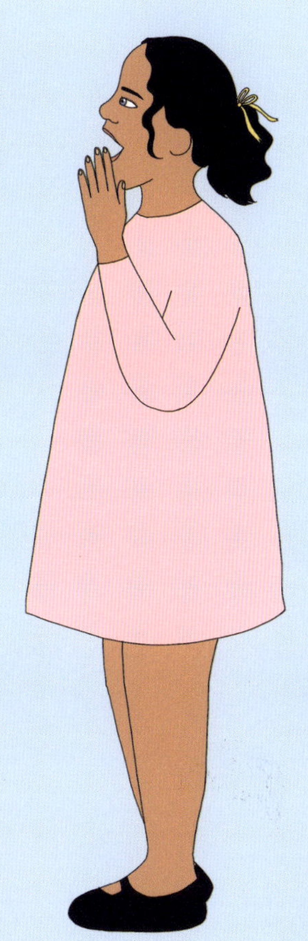
TO SPEAK, TO SHOUT, TO SING.

WE LEARN HOW TO MOVE...

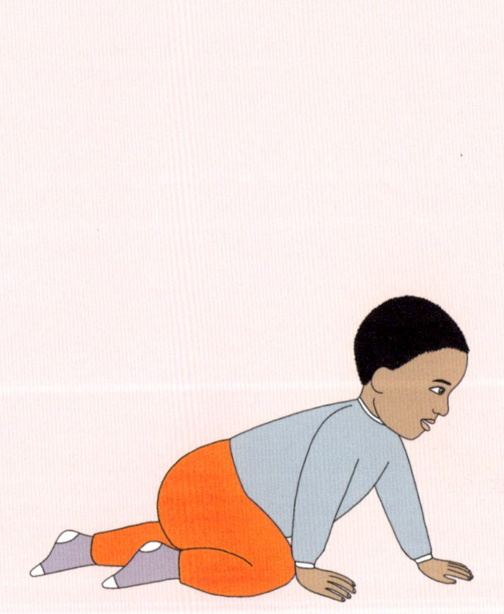

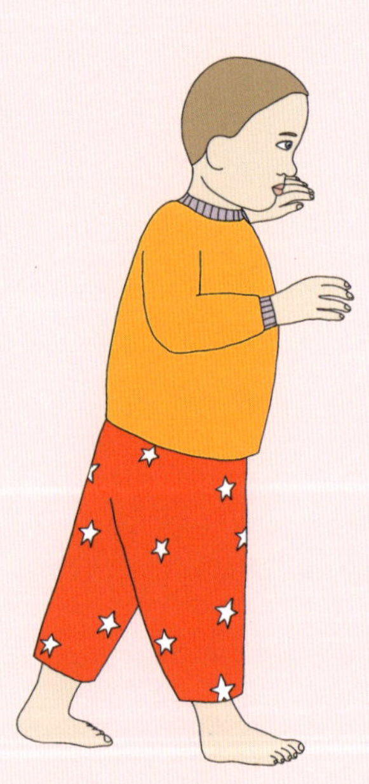

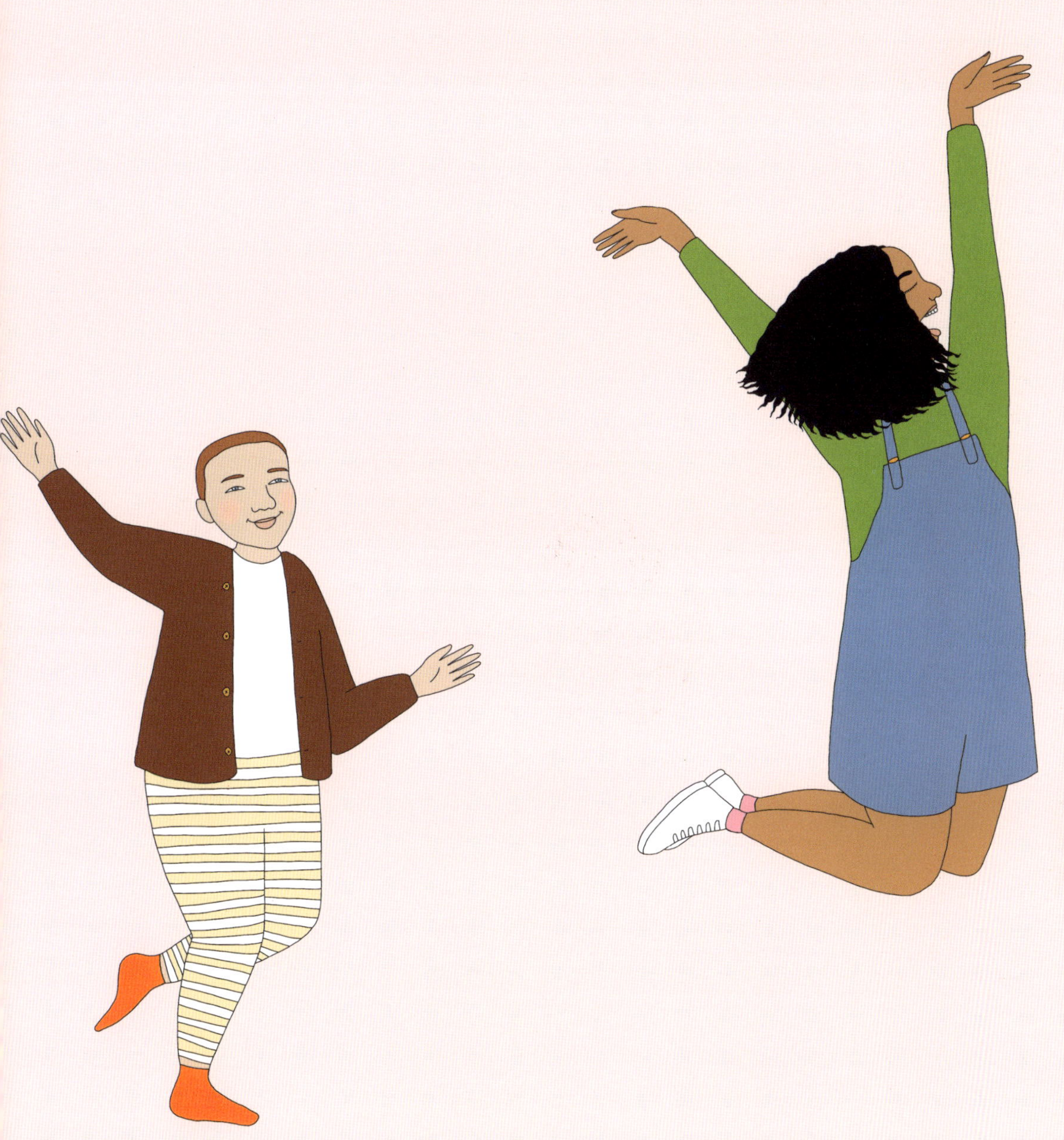

TO CRAWL, TO WALK, TO JUMP, TO DANCE.

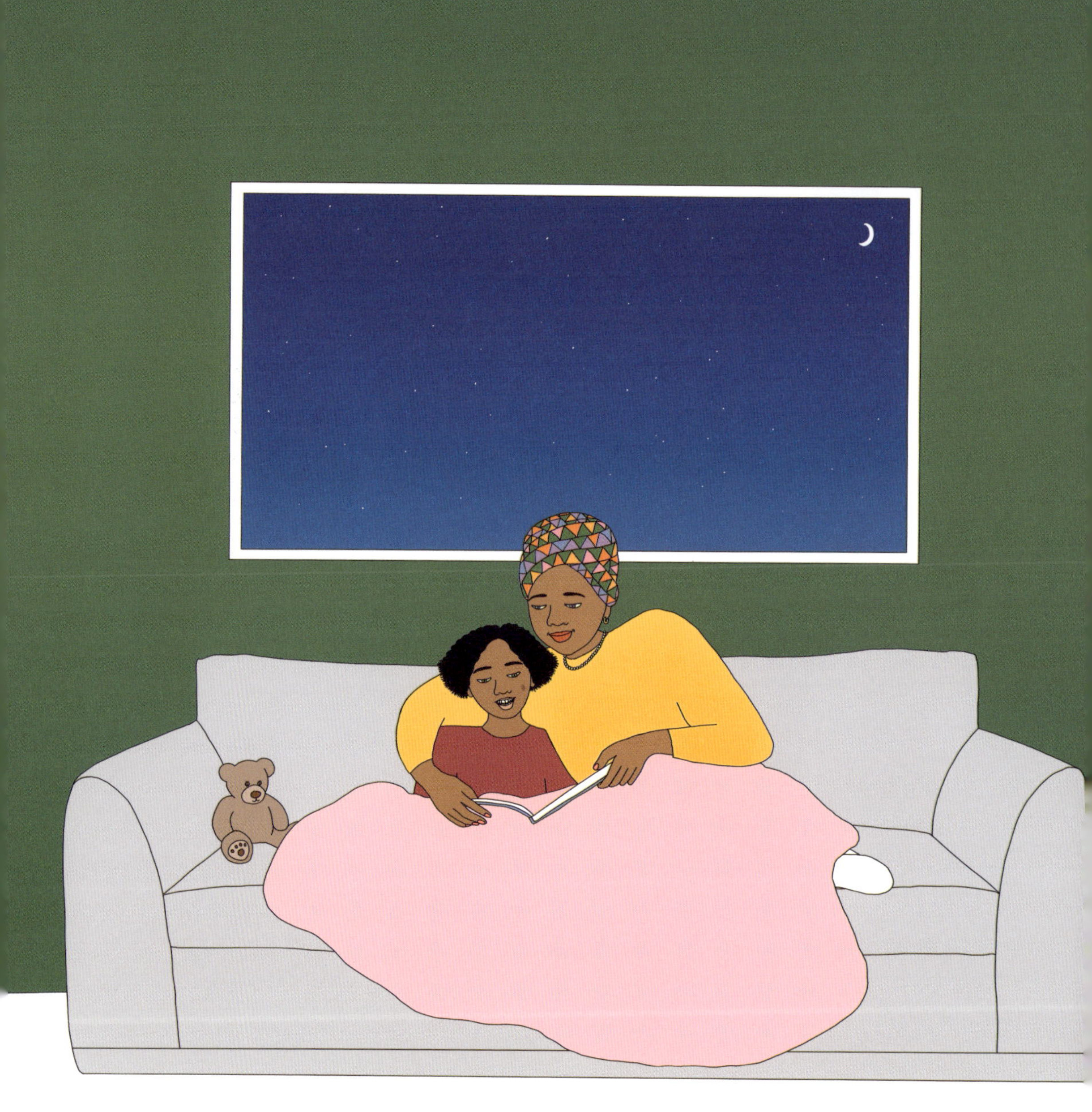

WE LEARN WHAT IT
FEELS LIKE TO BE LOVED

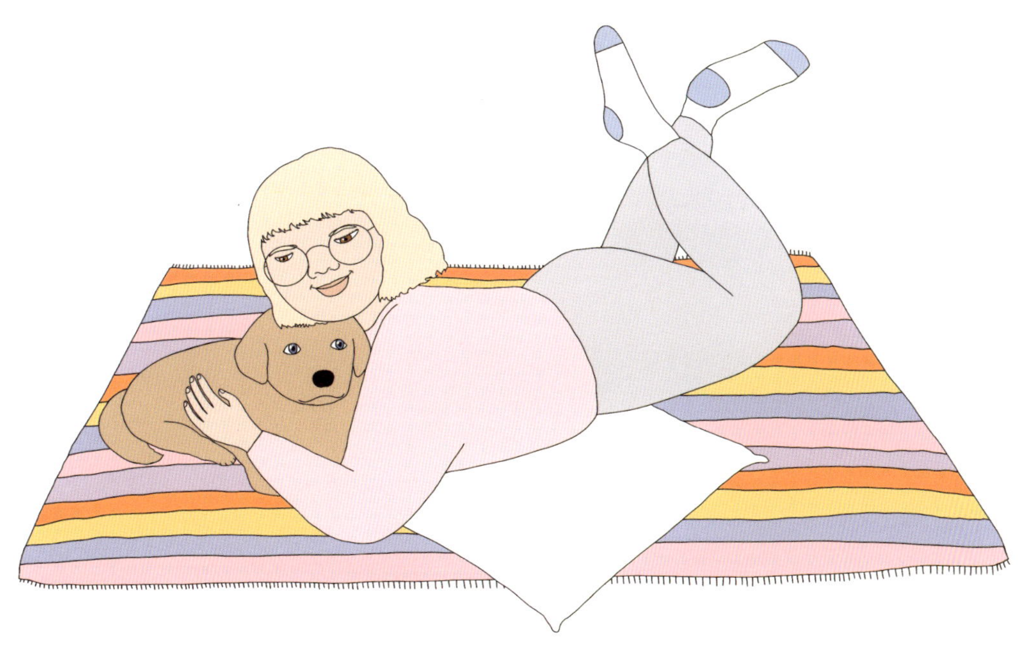

AND TO GIVE LOVE BACK.

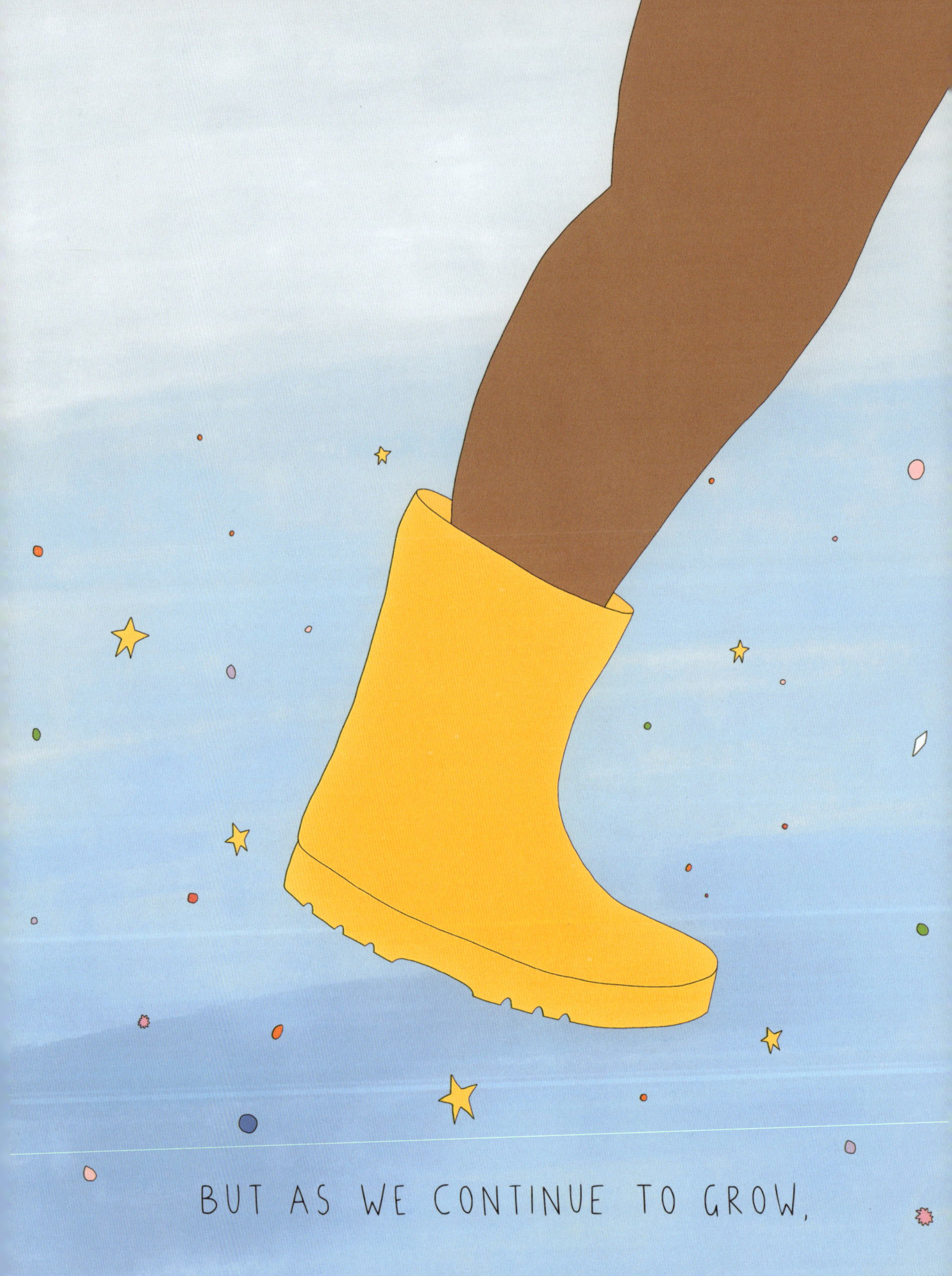

BUT AS WE CONTINUE TO GROW,

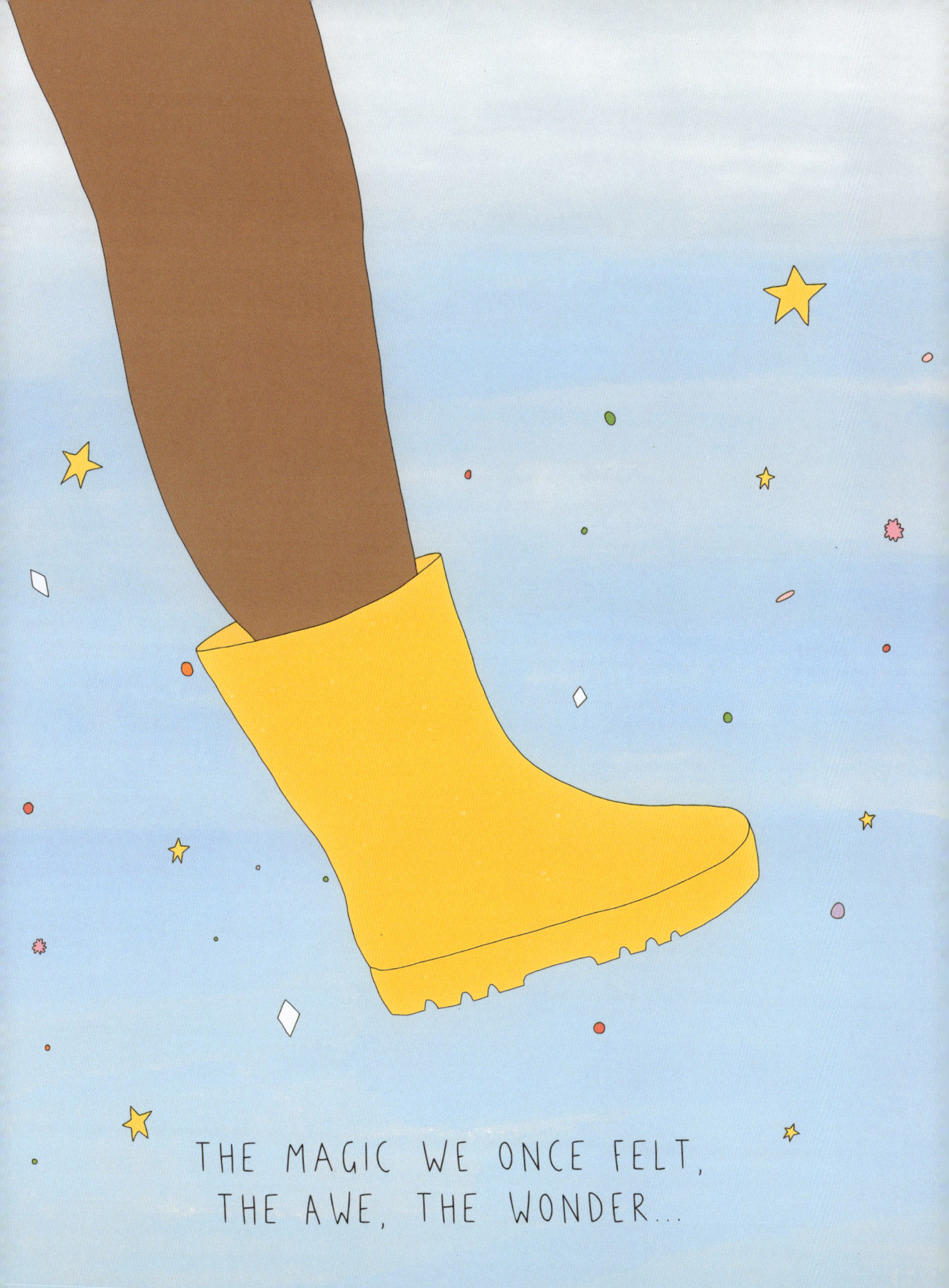
THE MAGIC WE ONCE FELT,
THE AWE, THE WONDER...

SEEMS TO SLIP AWAY...

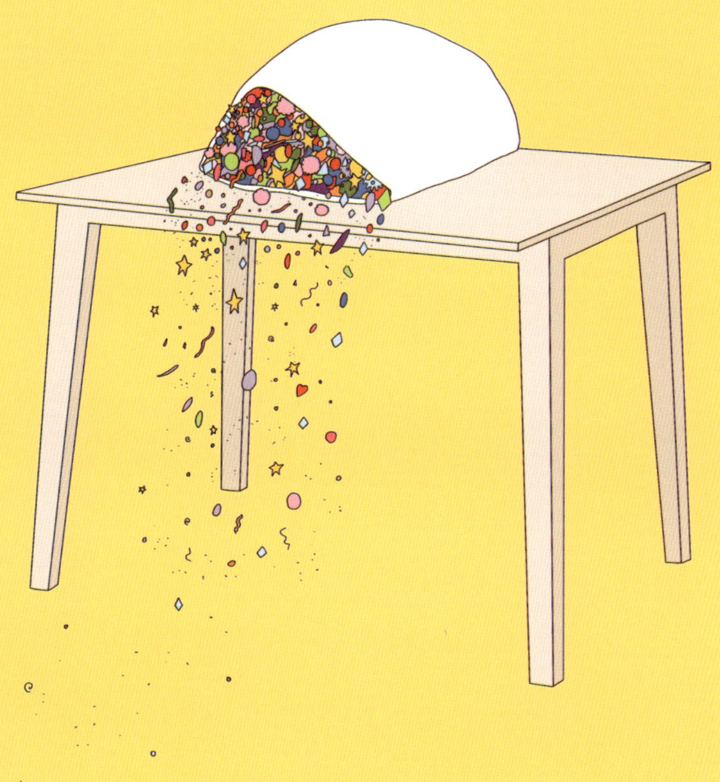

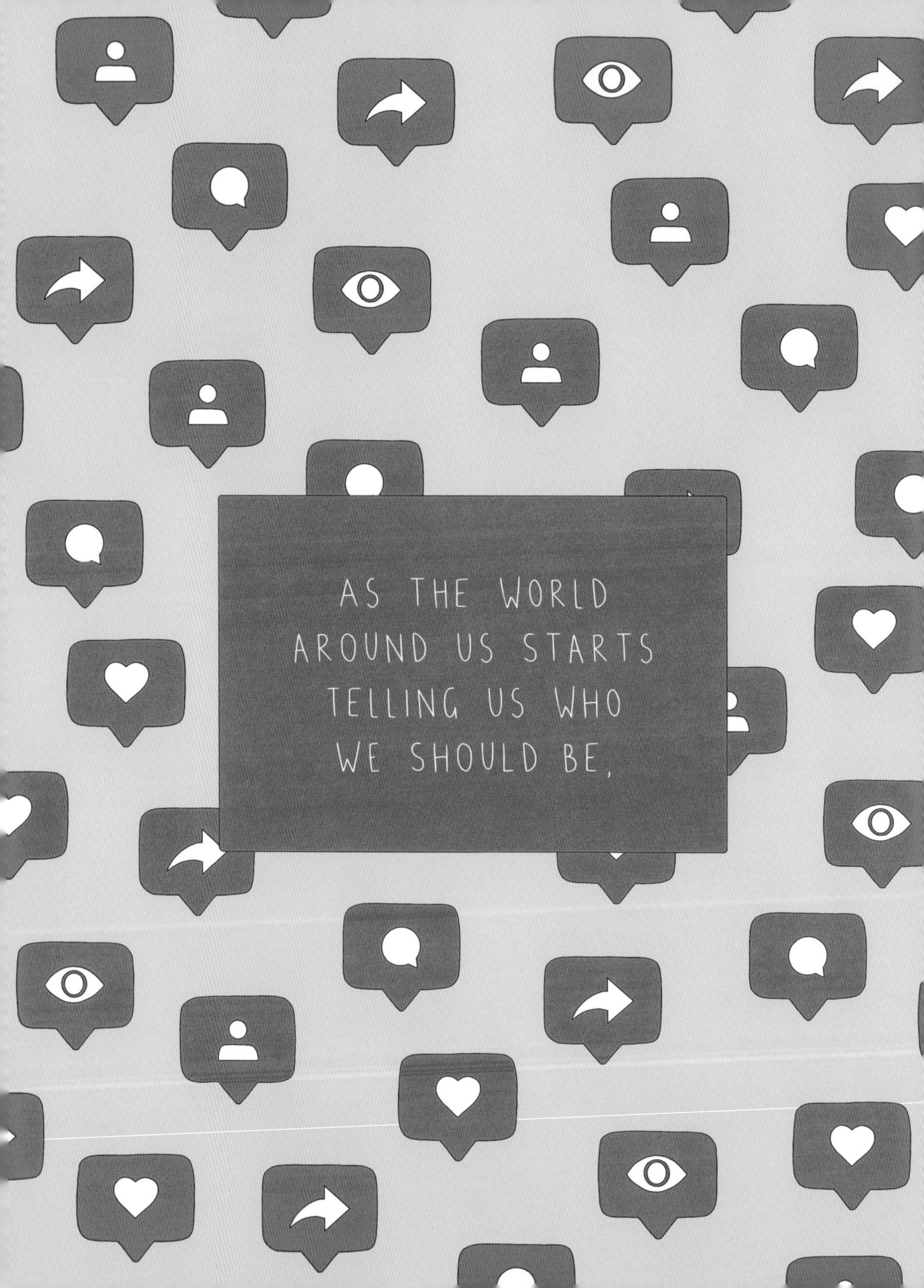
AS THE WORLD
AROUND US STARTS
TELLING US WHO
WE SHOULD BE,

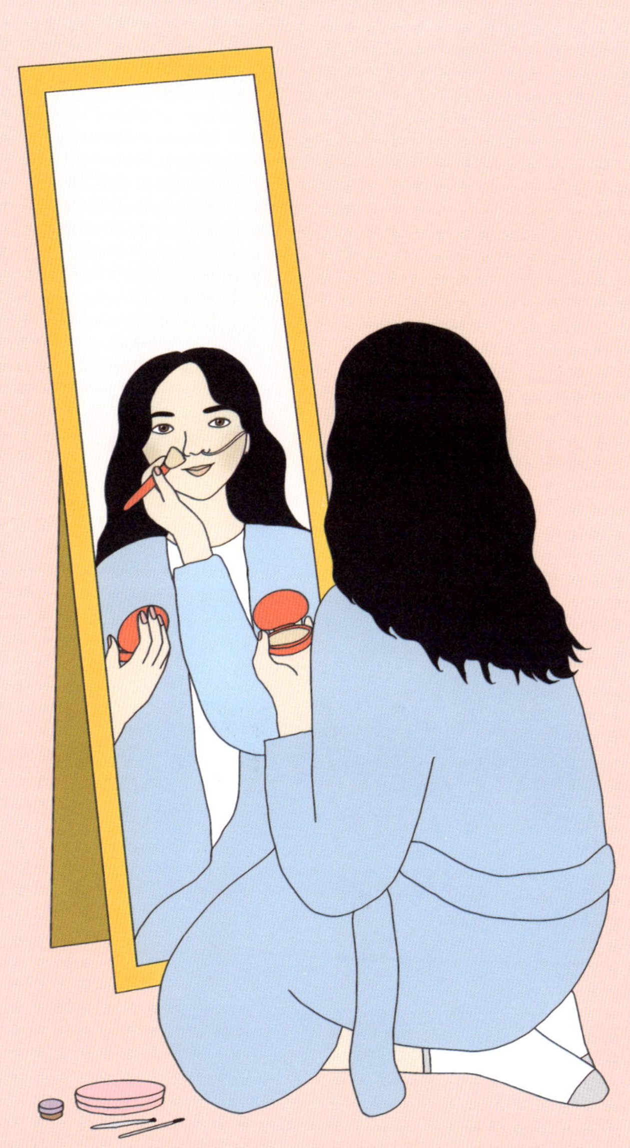

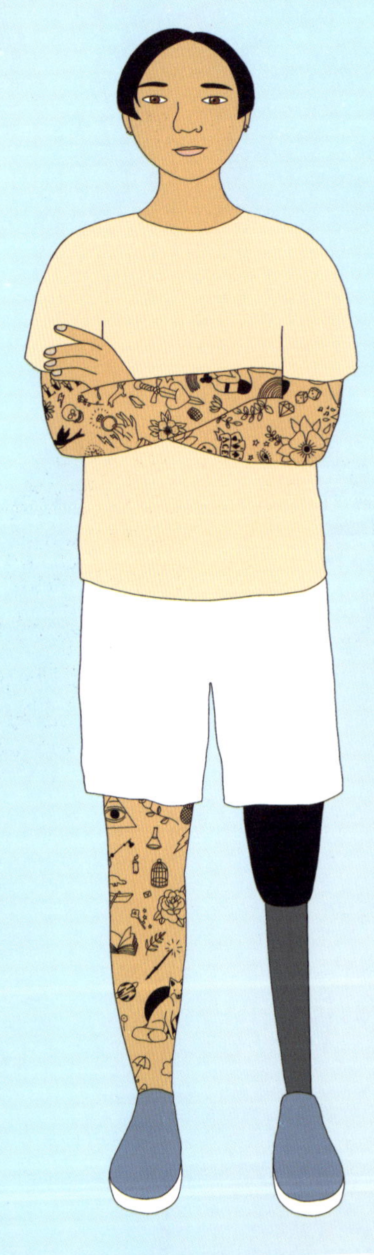

WHAT WE SHOULD LOOK LIKE,

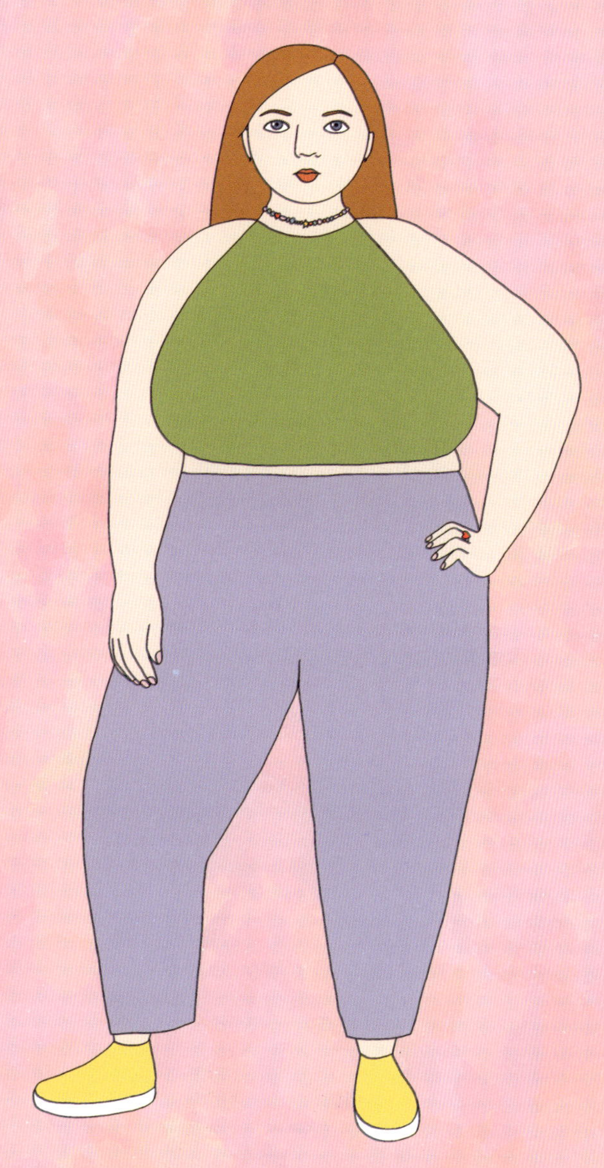

HOW WE SHOULD DRESS,

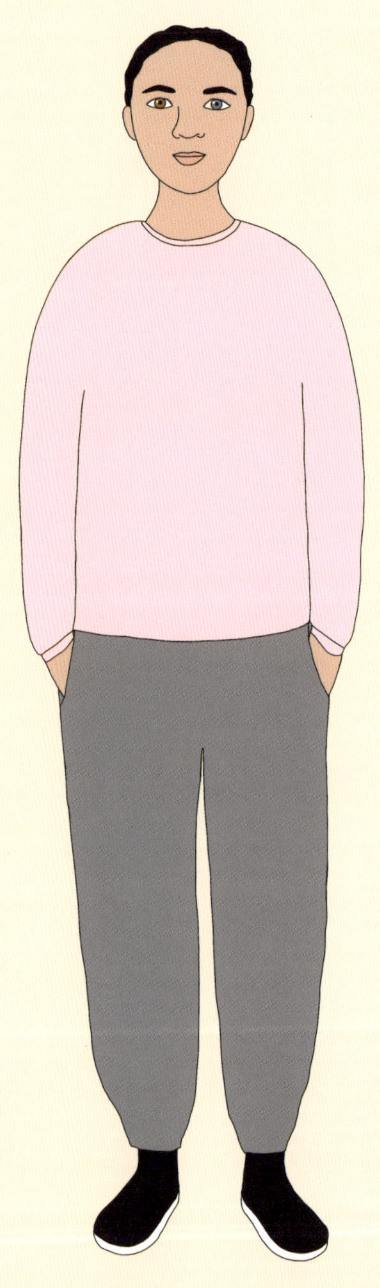

WHAT WE SHOULD SOUND LIKE,

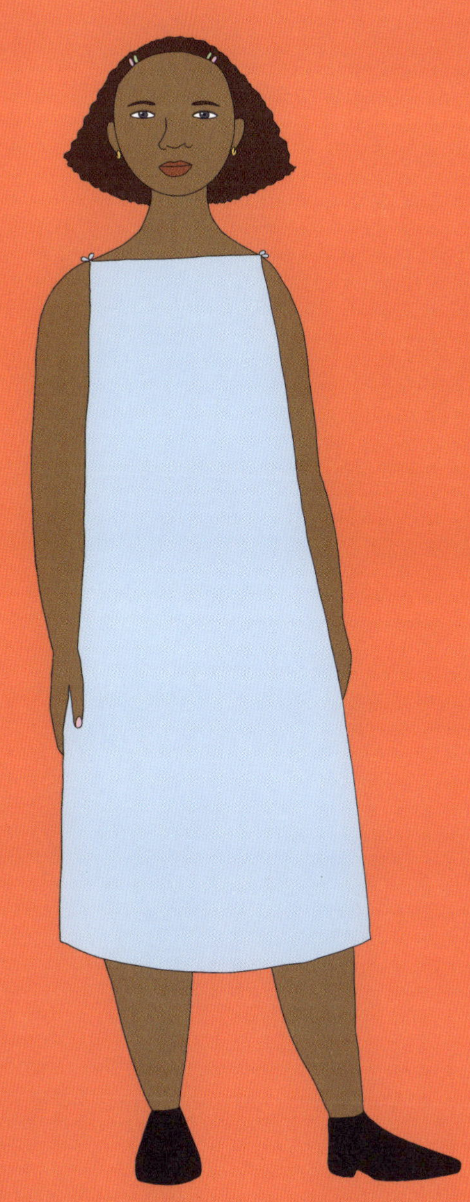

HOW WE SHOULD LIVE OUR LIVES.

THE MAGIC WE ONCE FELT IS REPLACED WITH ENDLESS

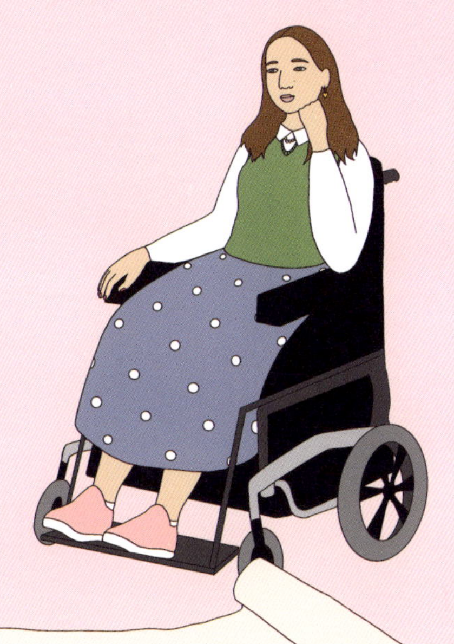

LISTS AND IMPOSSIBLE EXPECTATIONS.

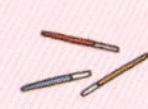

THE FOCUS SHIFTS FROM EVERYTHING OUR BODY CAN DO FOR US,

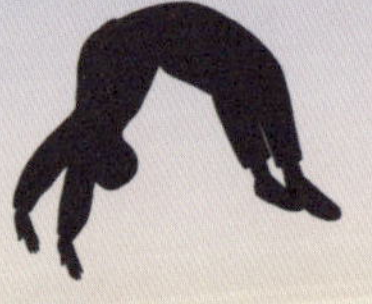

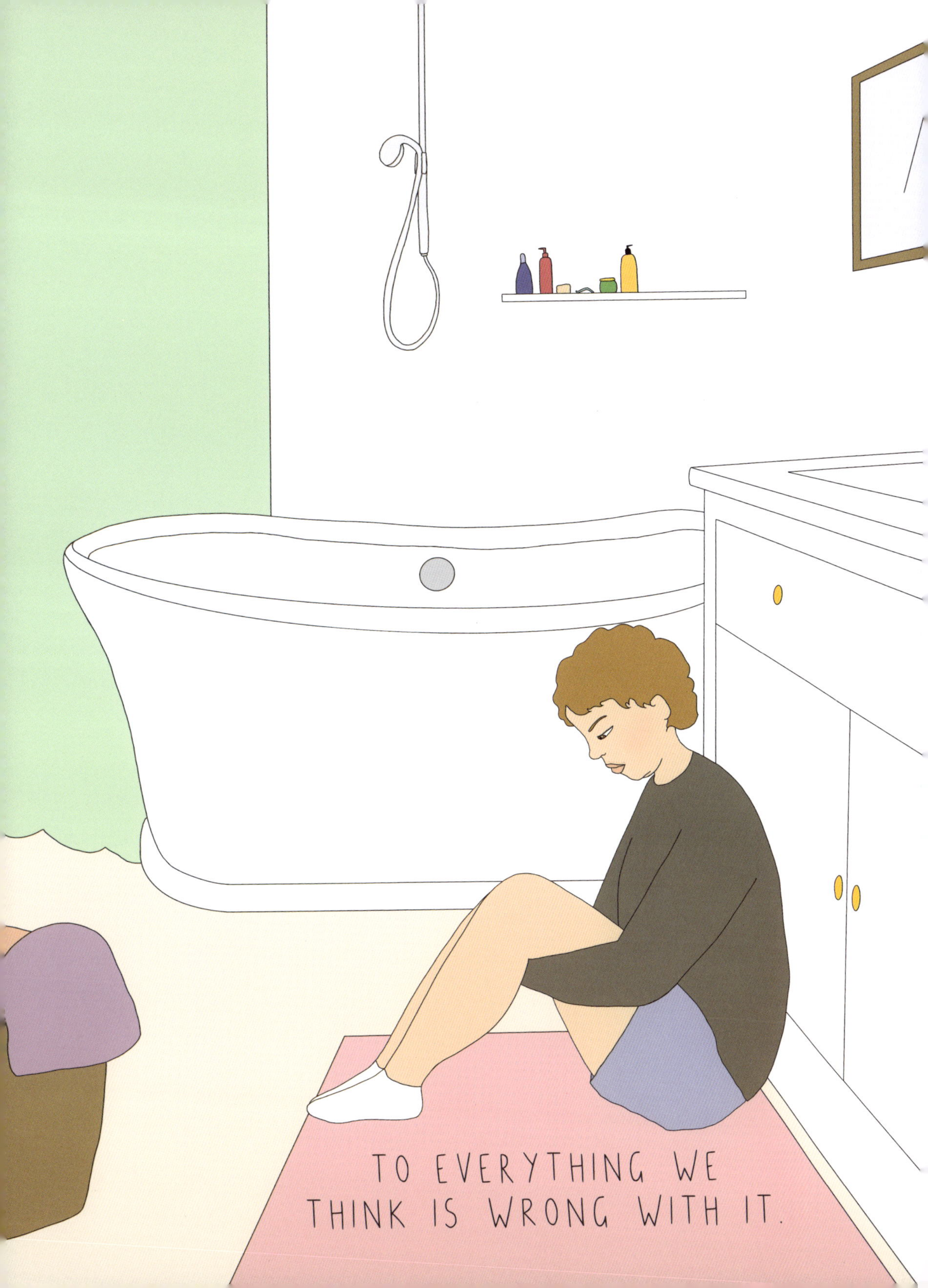
TO EVERYTHING WE
THINK IS WRONG WITH IT.

OF COURSE THE PATH TOWARDS
EMBRACING THE BODY
WE'RE IN ISN'T EASY.

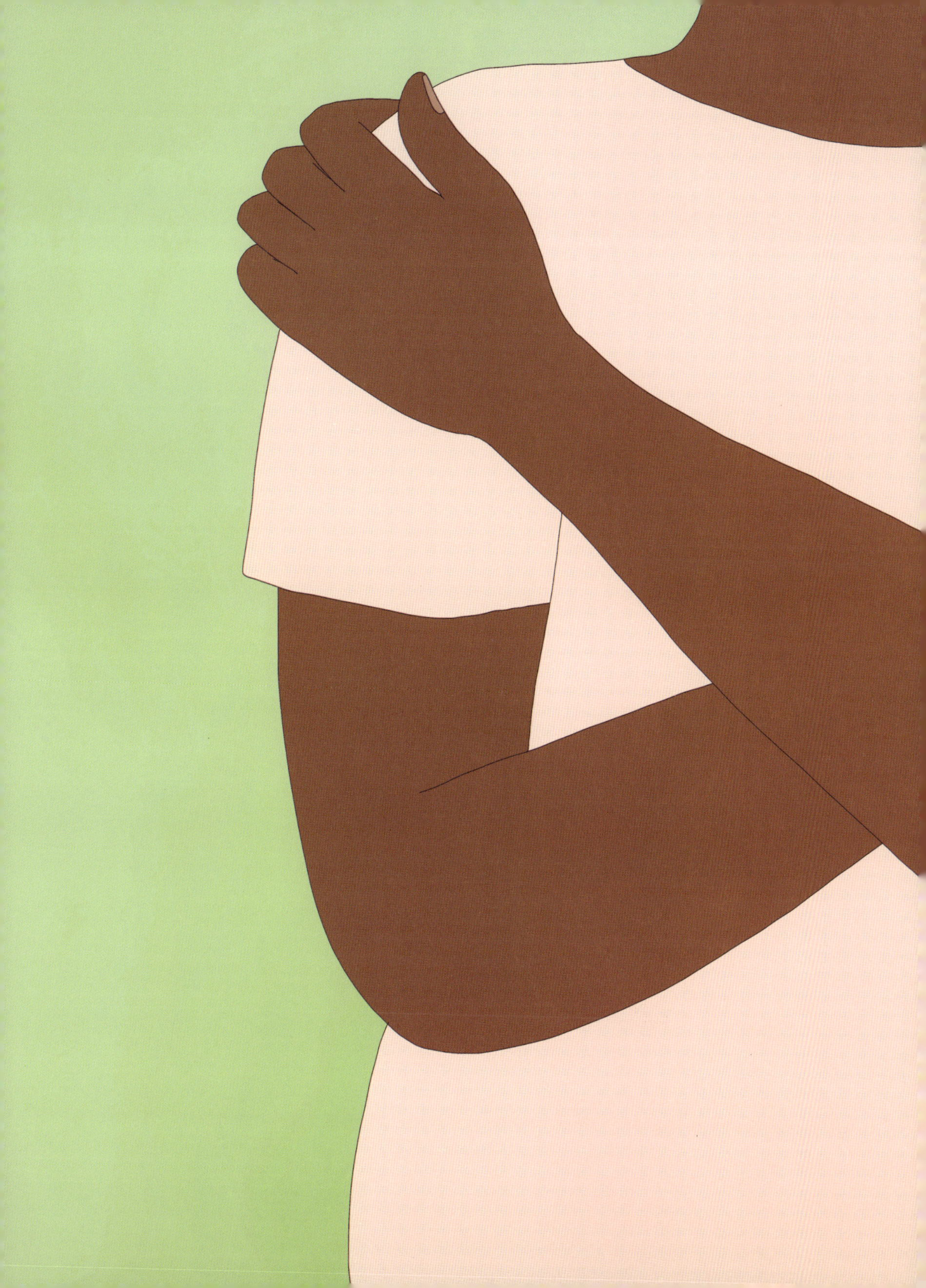

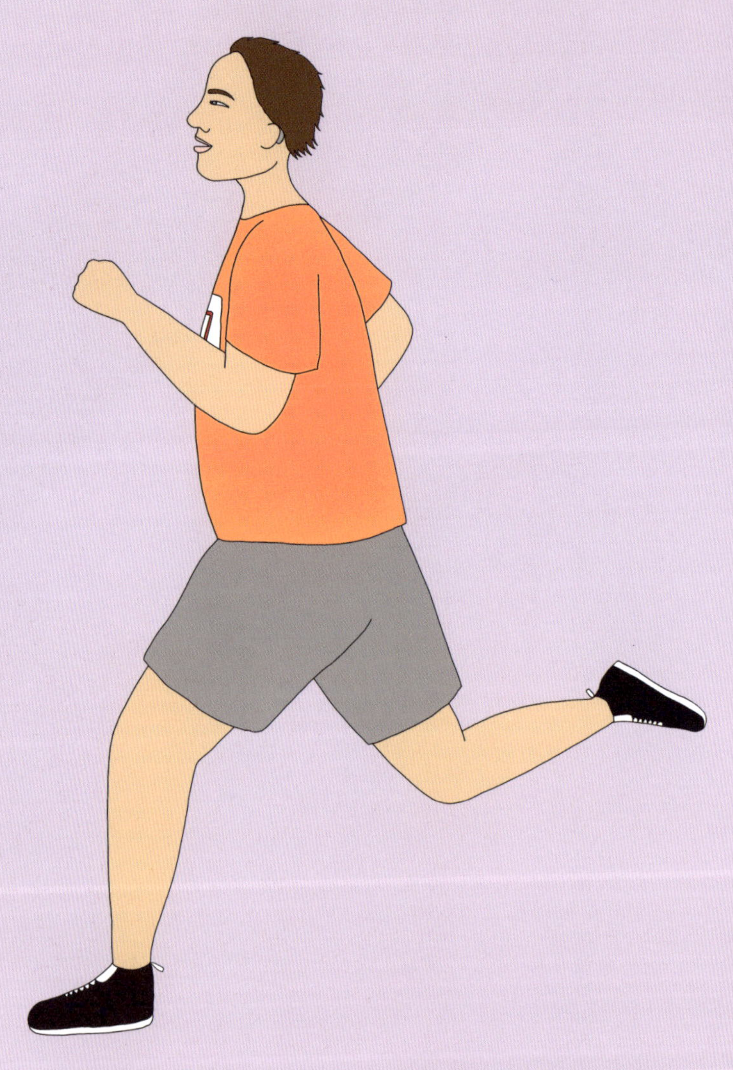

IT'S A LIFELONG JOURNEY
FULL OF SURPRISES,

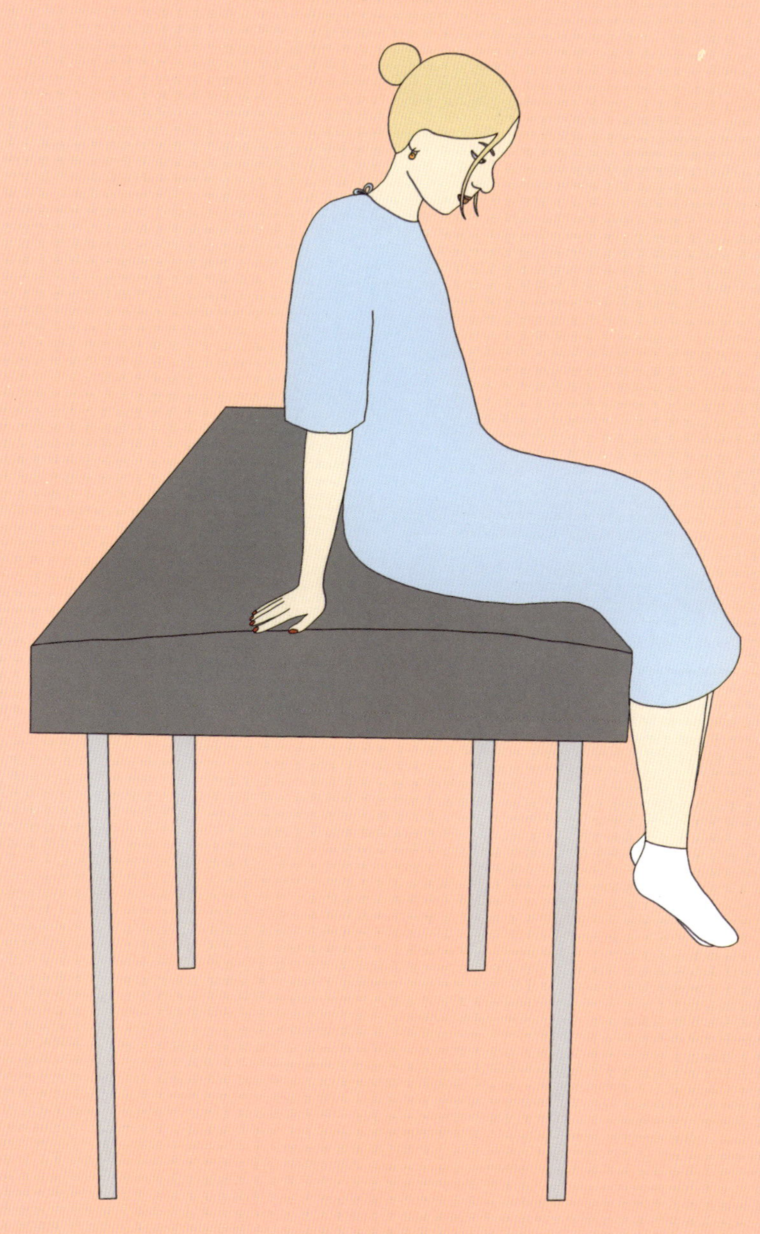

DISAPPOINTMENT,

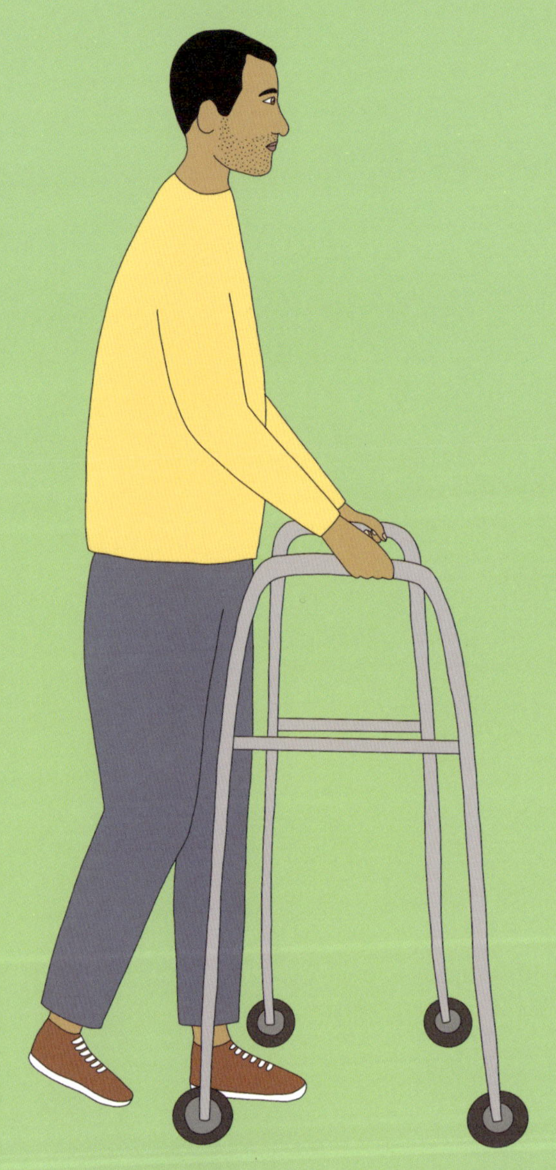

CHALLENGES,

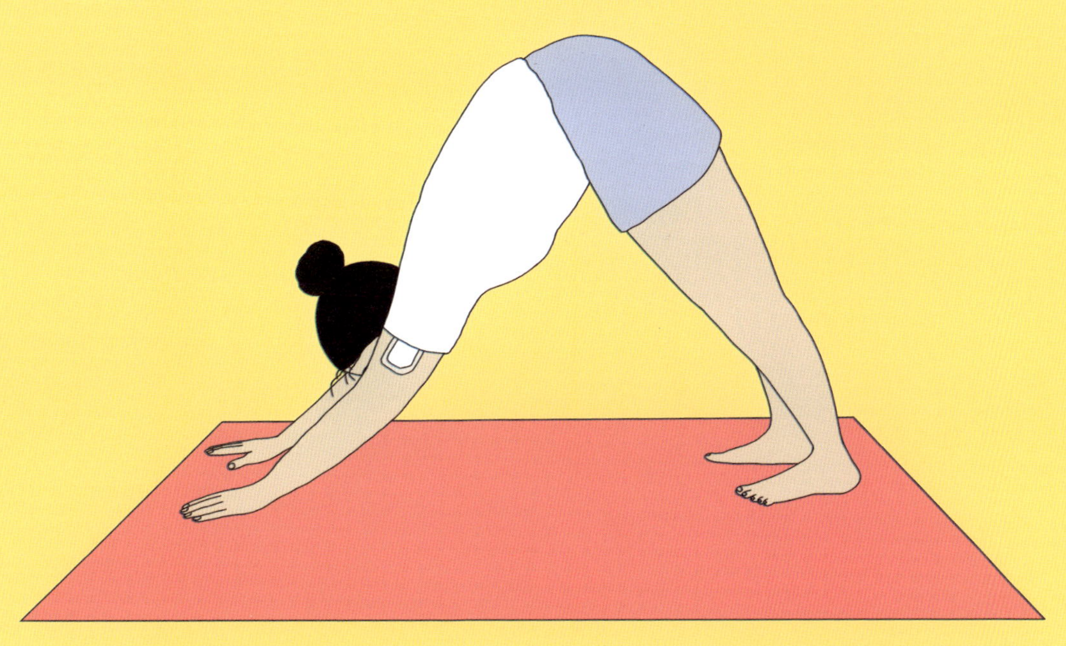

GROWTH.

AT TIMES YOU MIGHT FEEL YOUR BODY CHANGING IN WAYS YOU'RE NOT READY FOR...

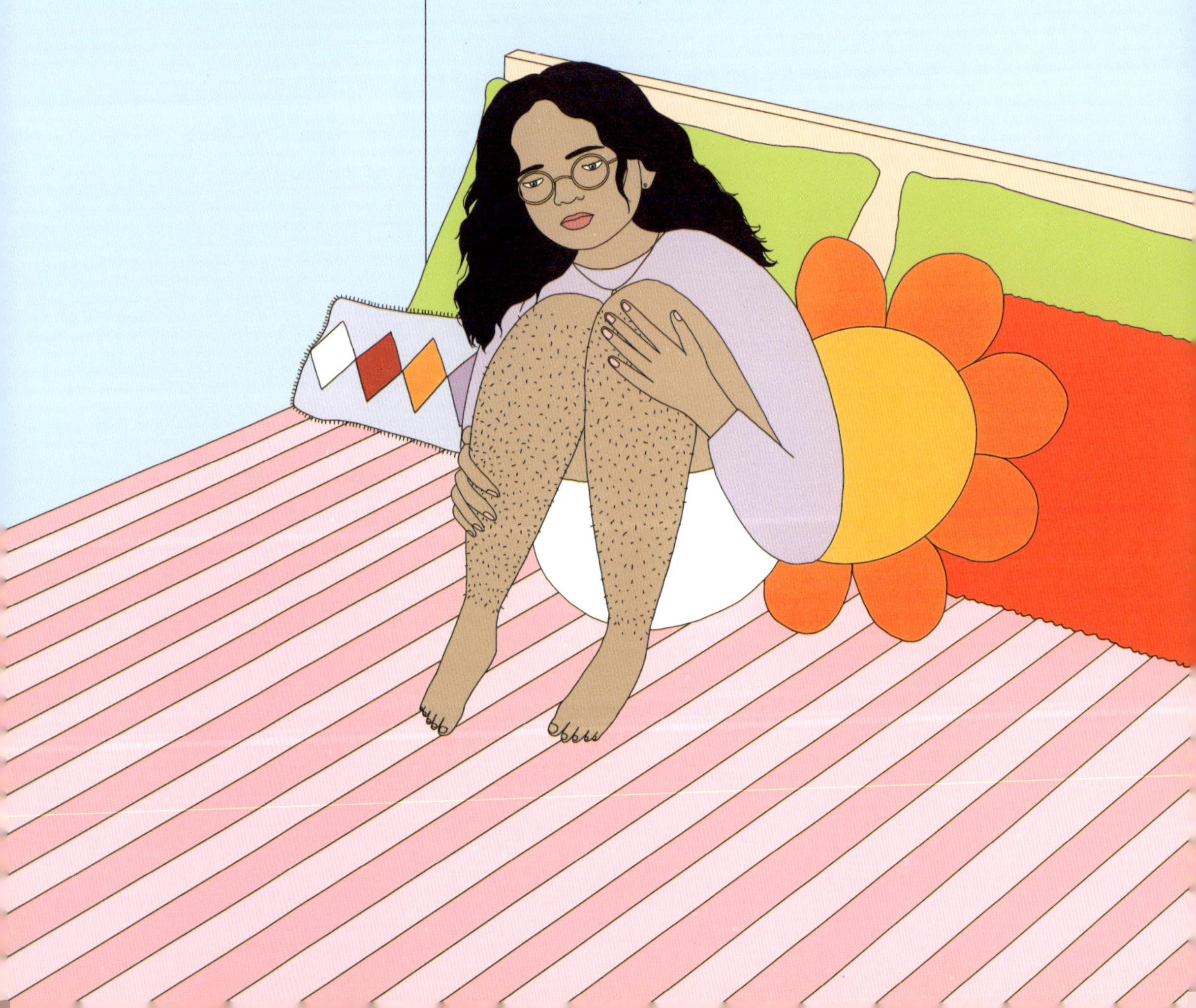

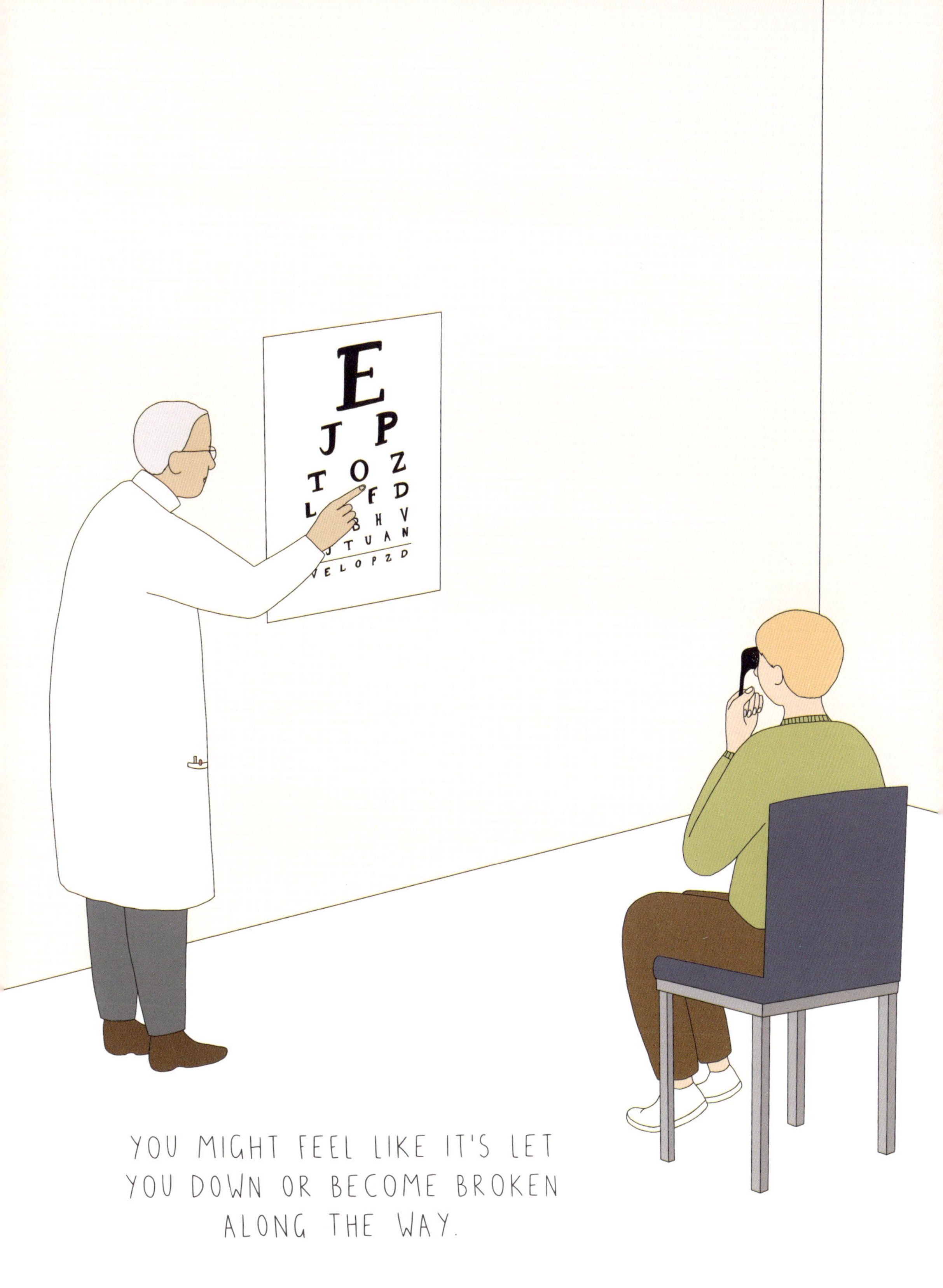
E
J P
T O Z
YOU MIGHT FEEL LIKE IT'S LET YOU DOWN OR BECOME BROKEN ALONG THE WAY.

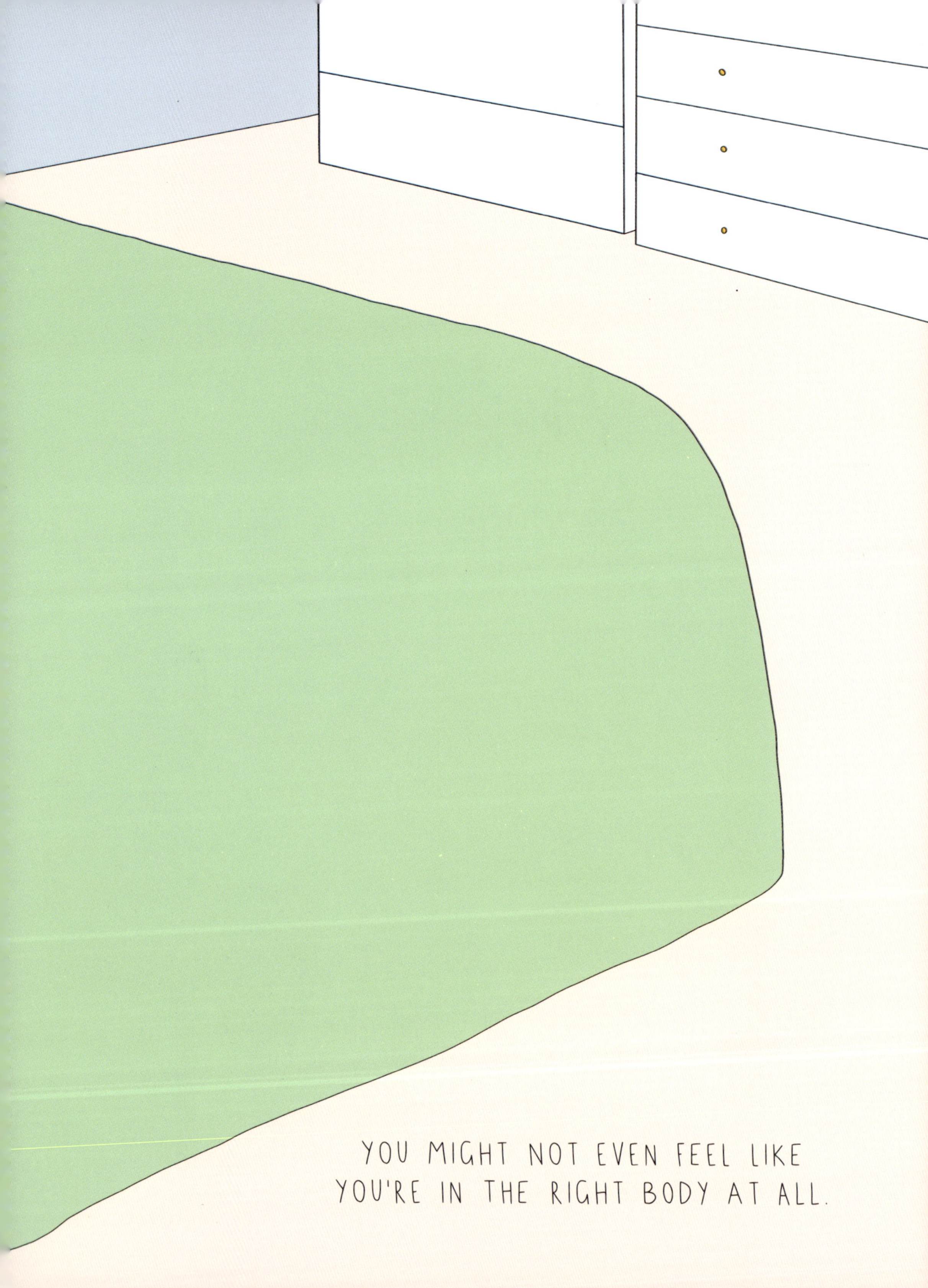
YOU MIGHT NOT EVEN FEEL LIKE
YOU'RE IN THE RIGHT BODY AT ALL.

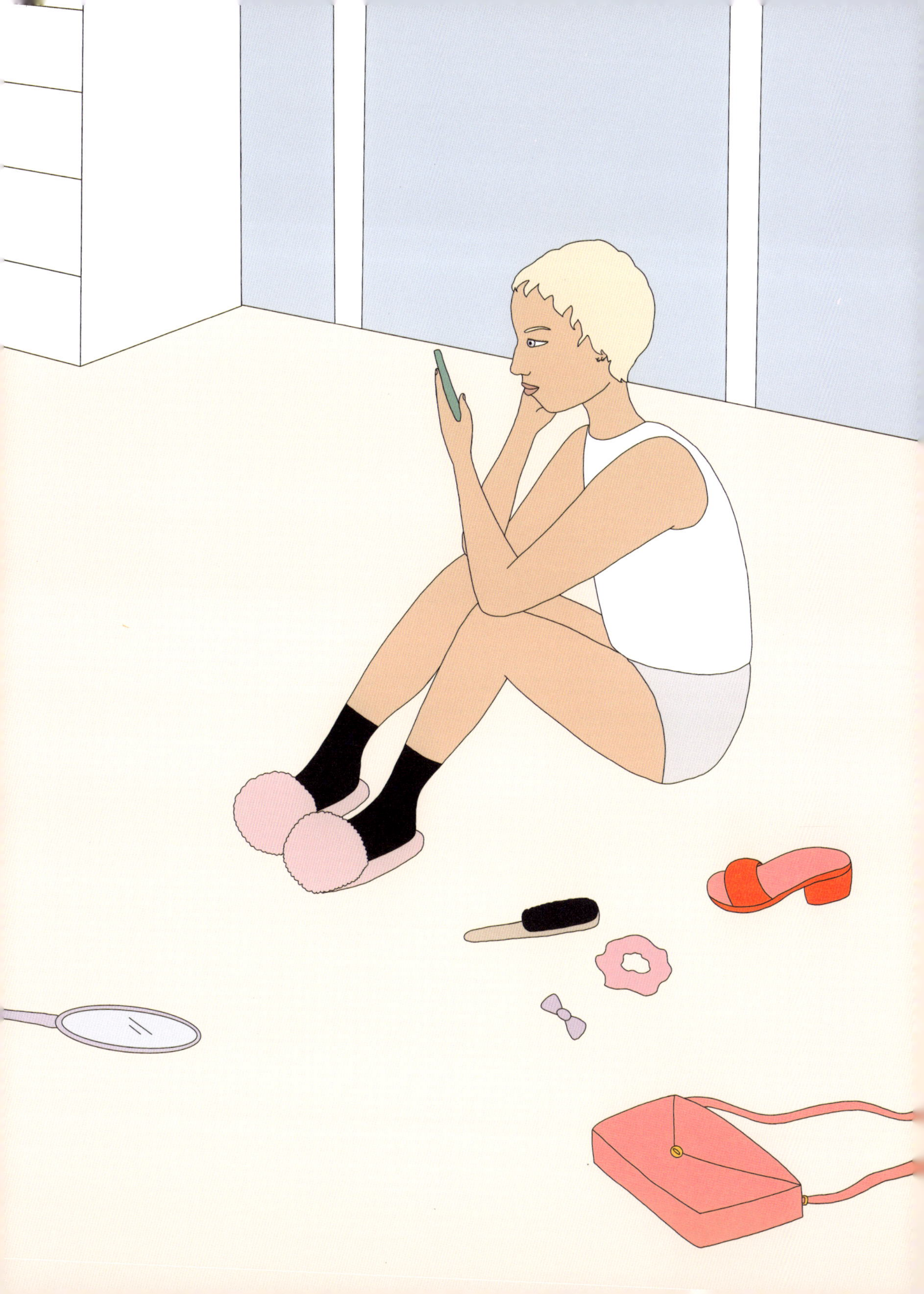

LEAN INTO THAT UNCERTAINTY,
THAT DISCOMFORT.
LET YOURSELF SIT WITH IT.

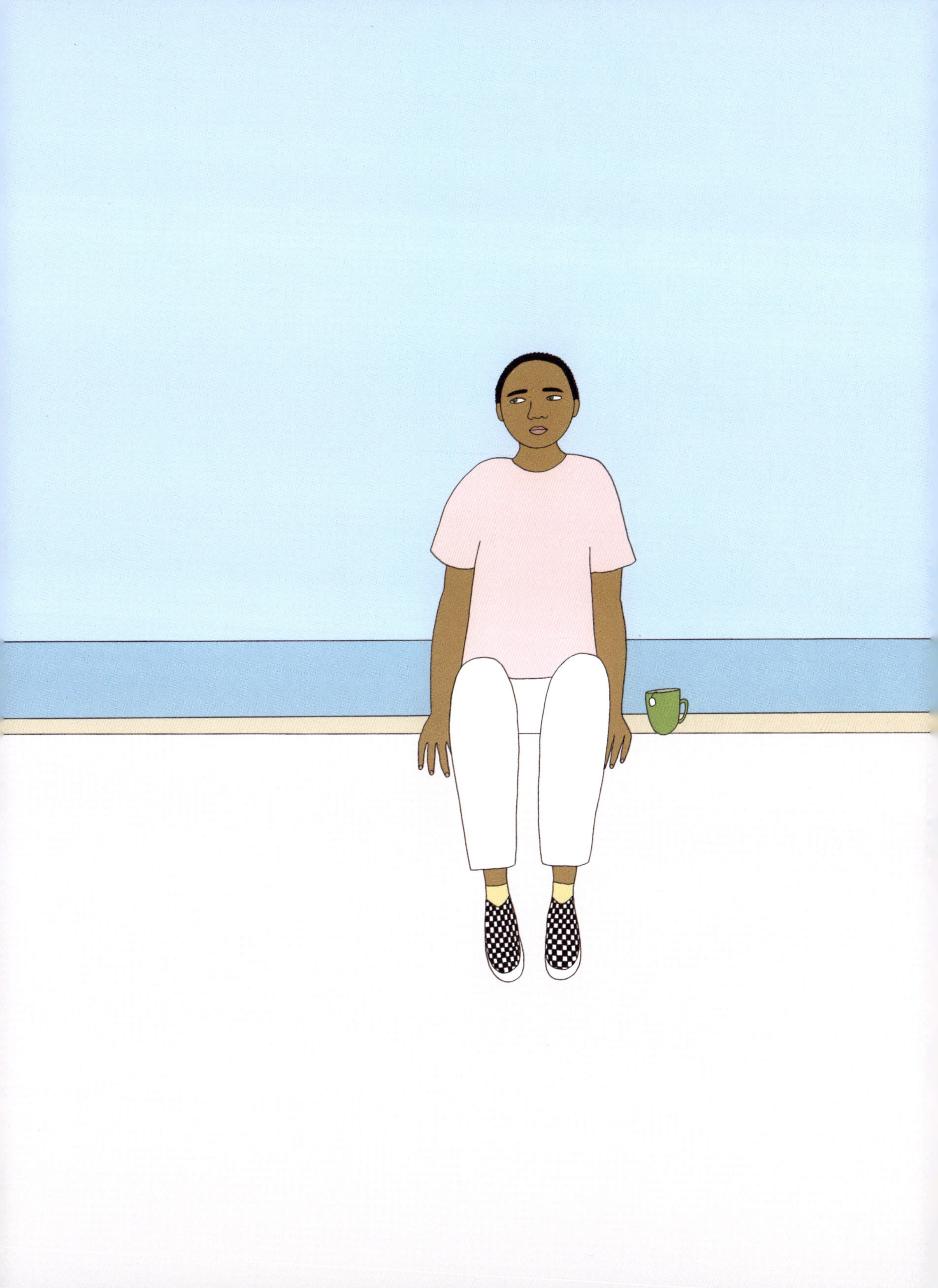

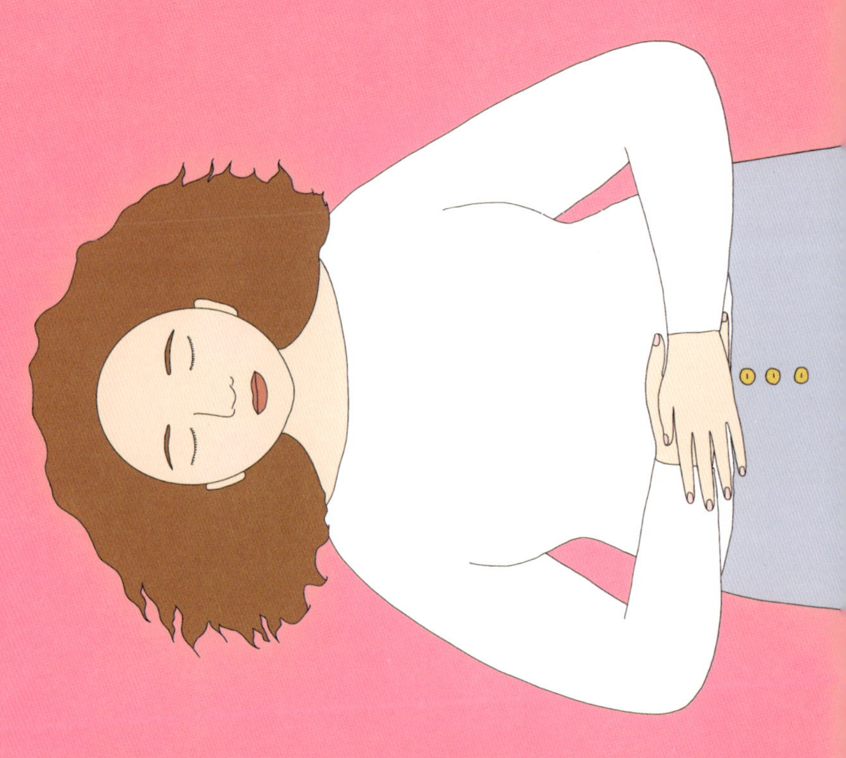

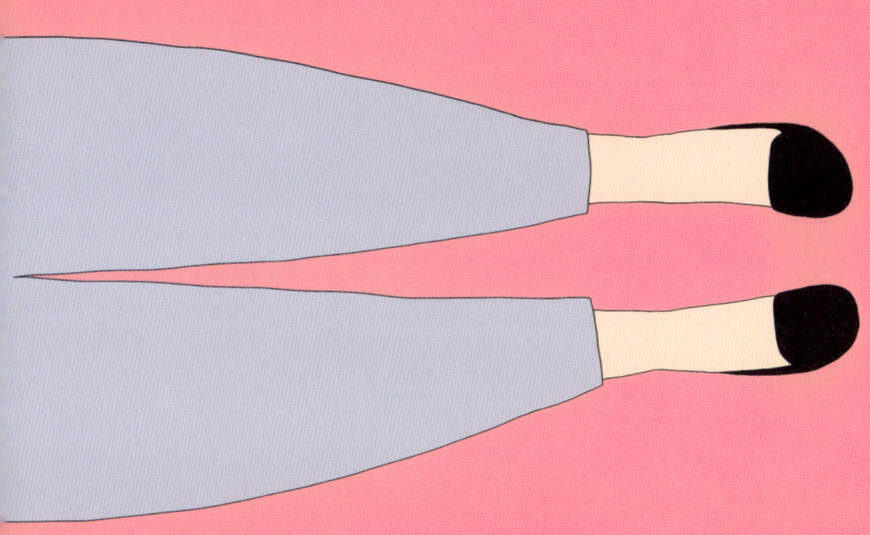

LISTEN TO YOUR BODY.

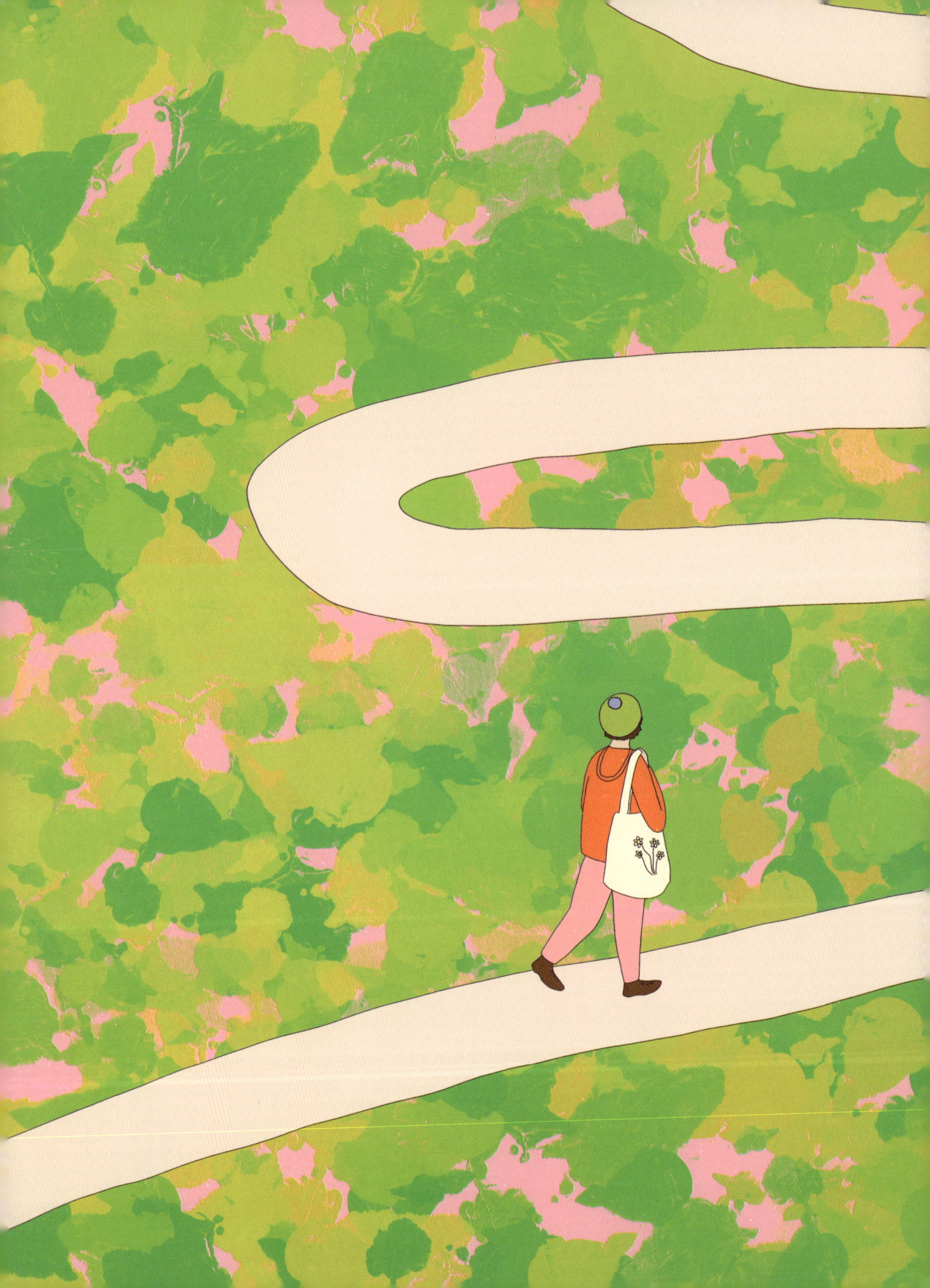

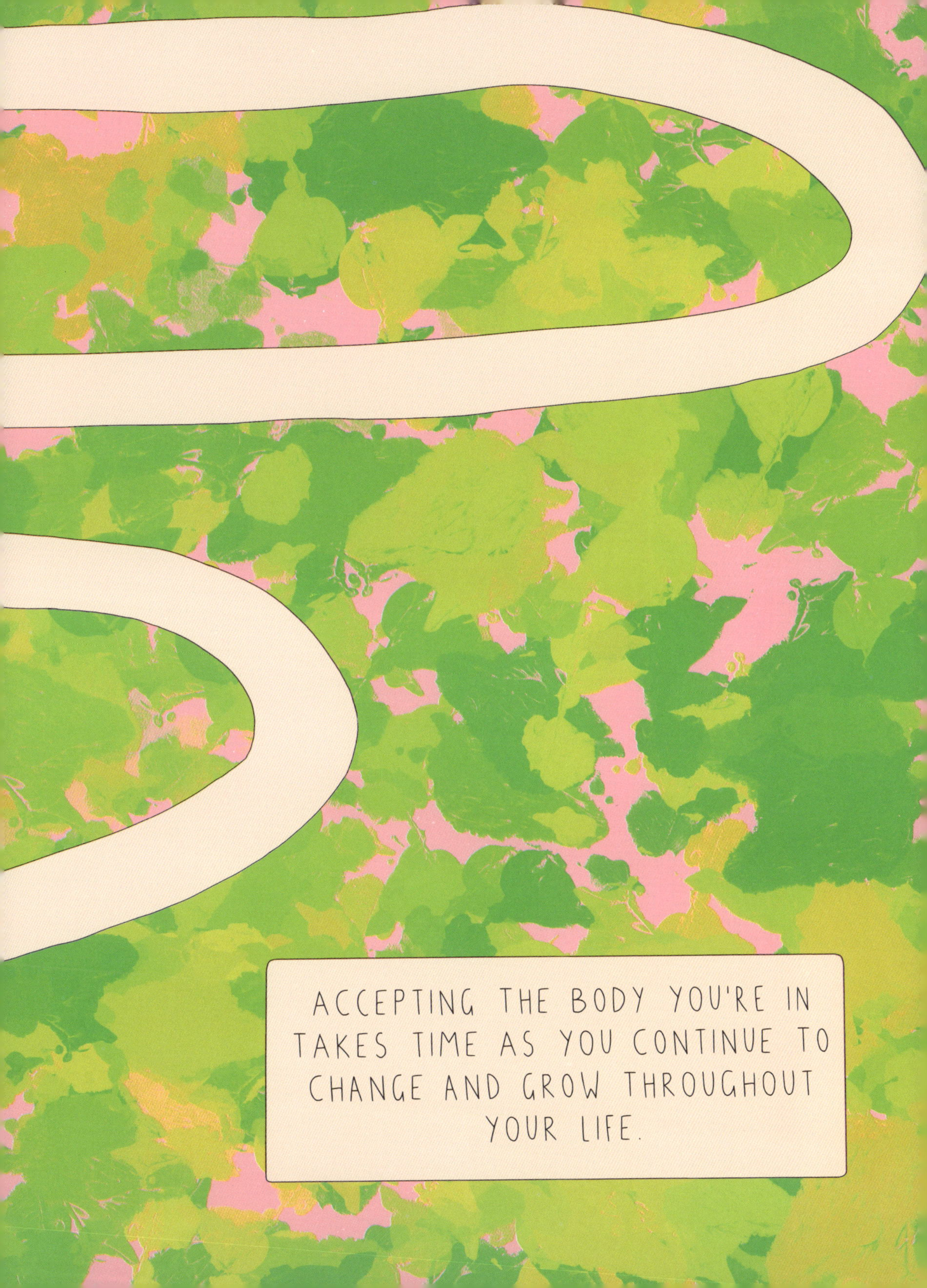
ACCEPTING THE BODY YOU'RE IN TAKES TIME AS YOU CONTINUE TO CHANGE AND GROW THROUGHOUT YOUR LIFE.

THE GOAL ISN'T TO LOVE EVERY SINGLE INCH OF YOUR BODY – THAT'S NOT REALISTIC.

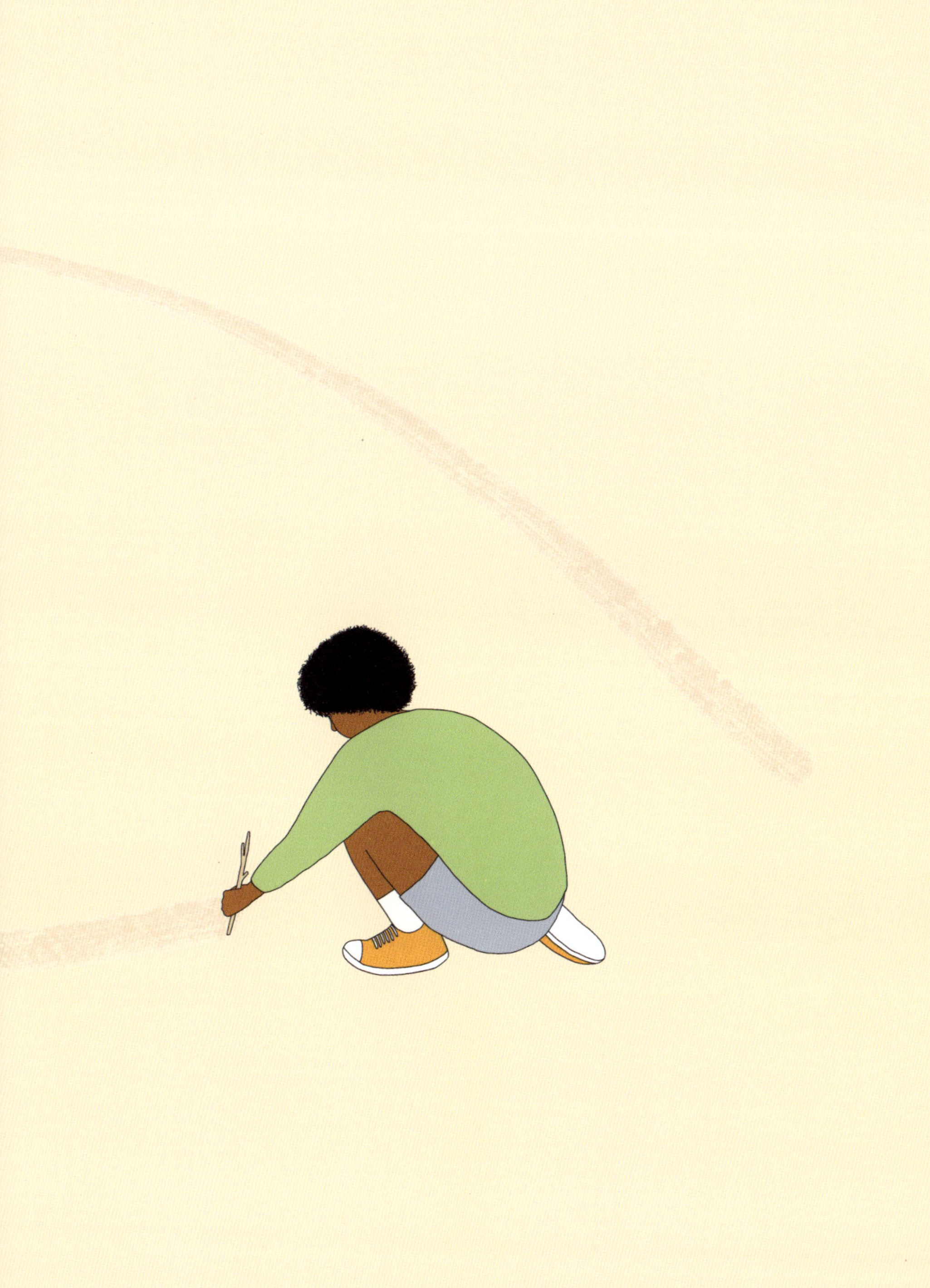

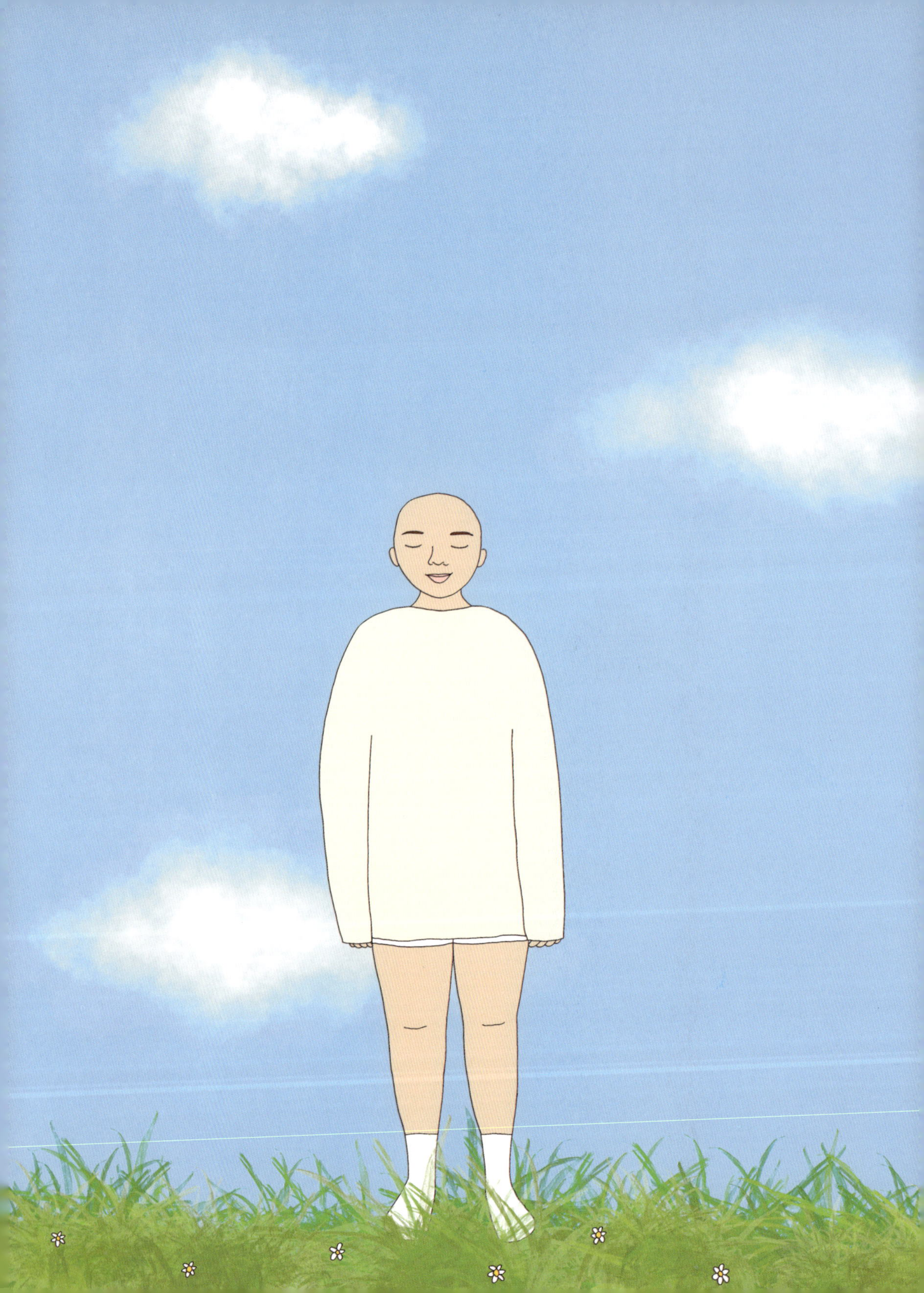

THE GOAL IS TO REACH A PLACE OF ACCEPTANCE AND PEACE WITH THE SKIN YOU'RE IN.

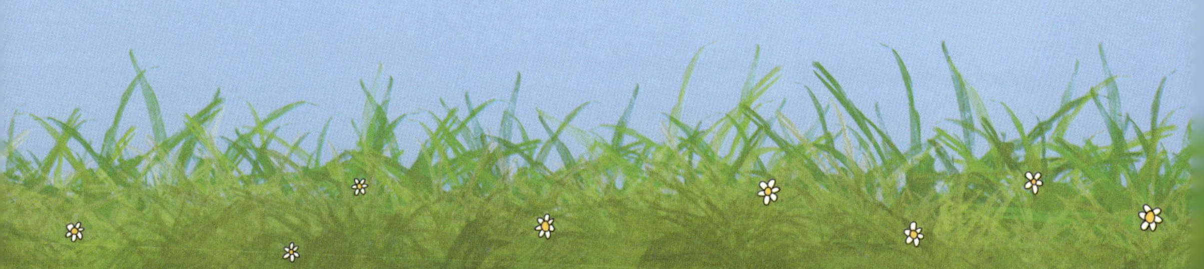

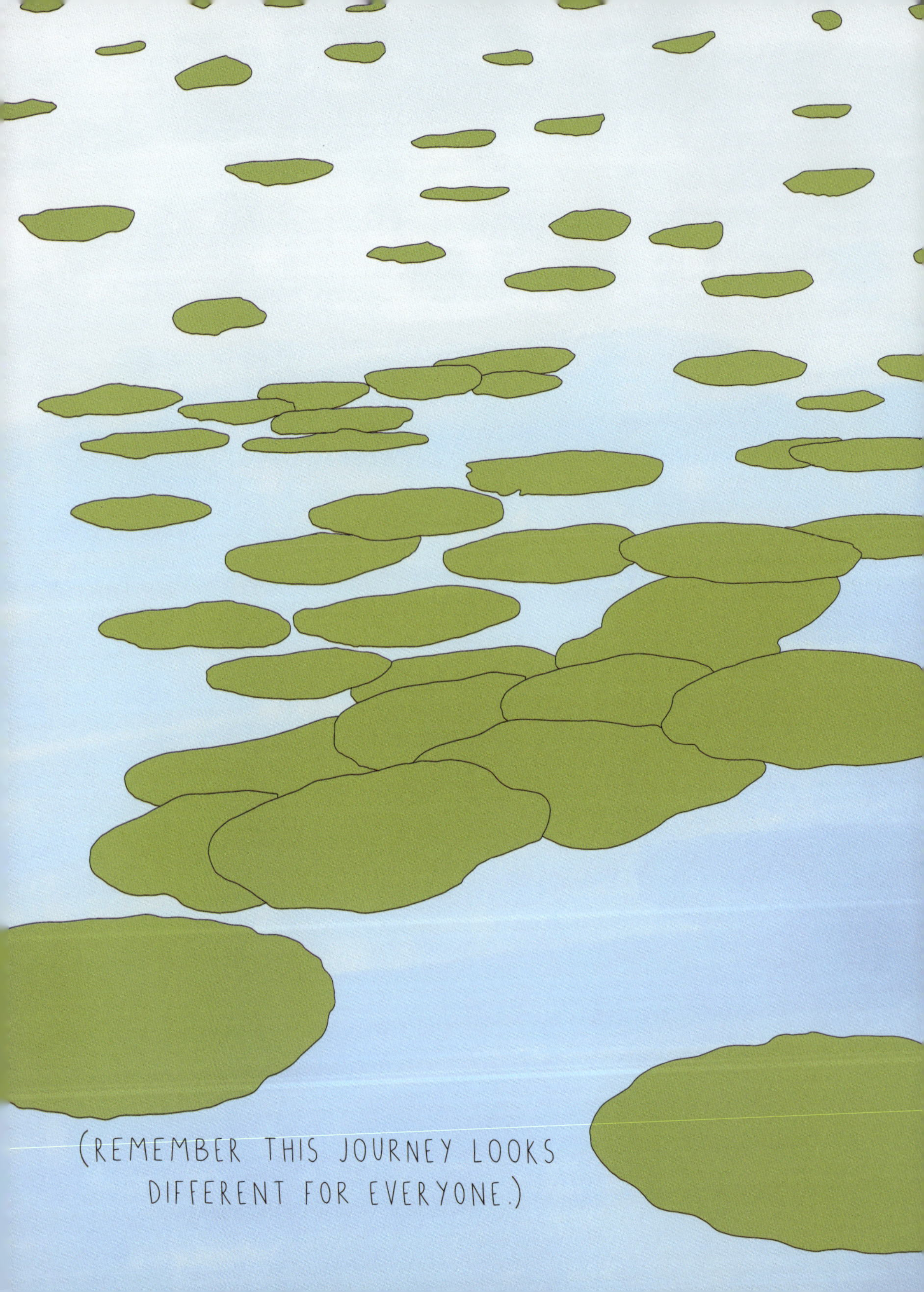
(REMEMBER THIS JOURNEY LOOKS
DIFFERENT FOR EVERYONE.)

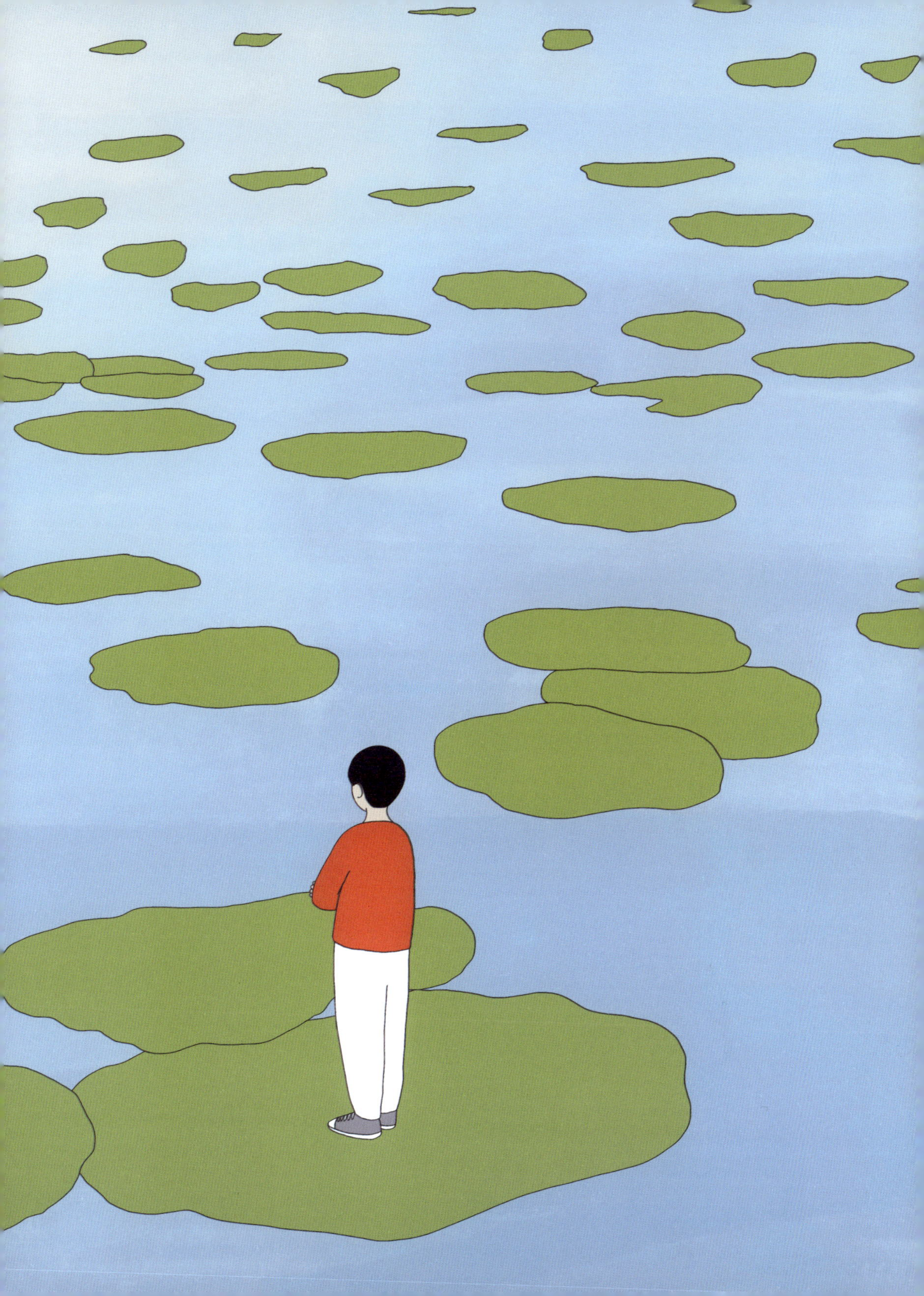

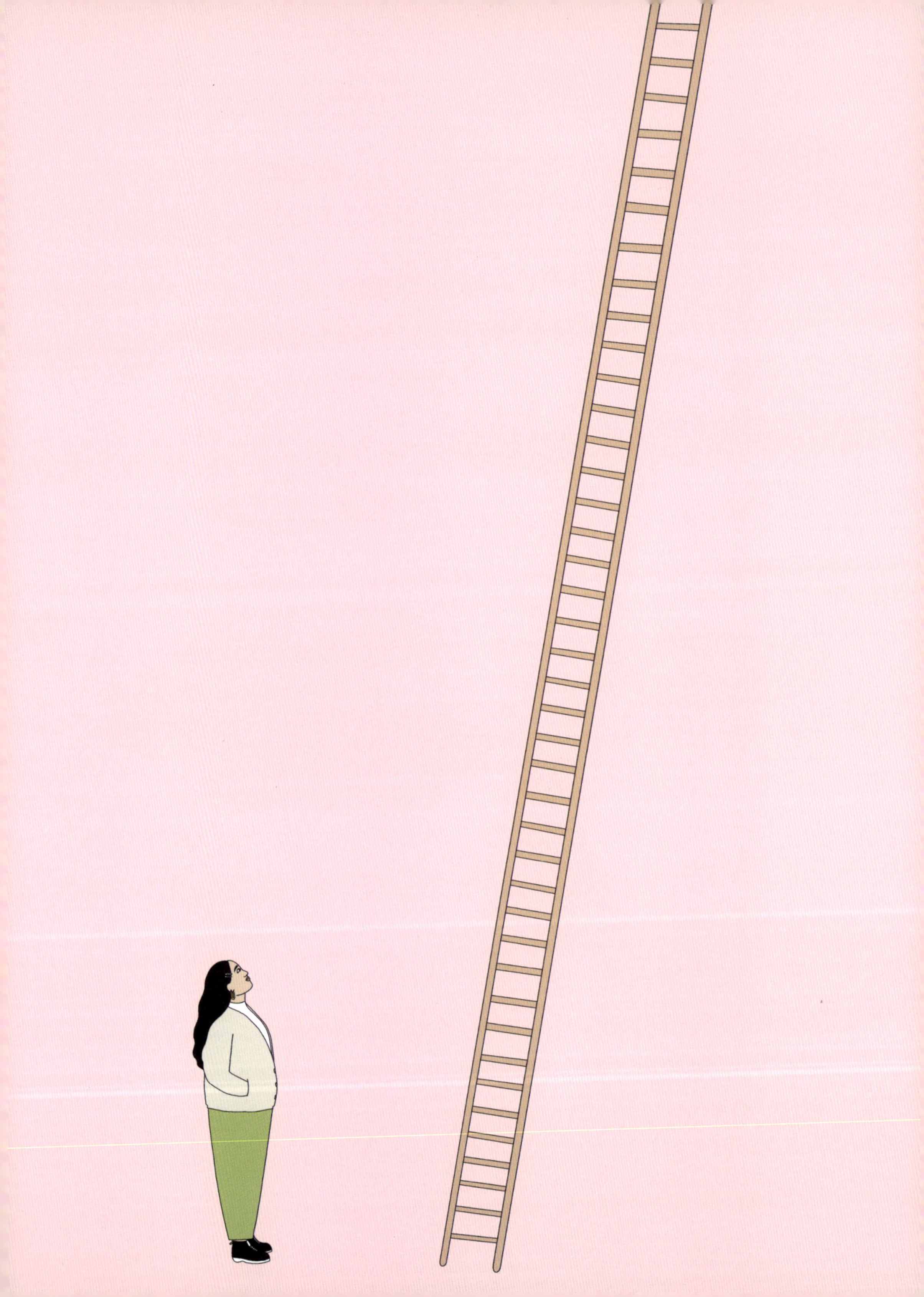

IT TAKES TIME TO BUILD
CONFIDENCE WITHIN
OURSELVES.

SOME DAYS THAT
CONFIDENCE COMES EASILY;
OTHER DAYS IT TAKES
A LITTLE MORE WORK.

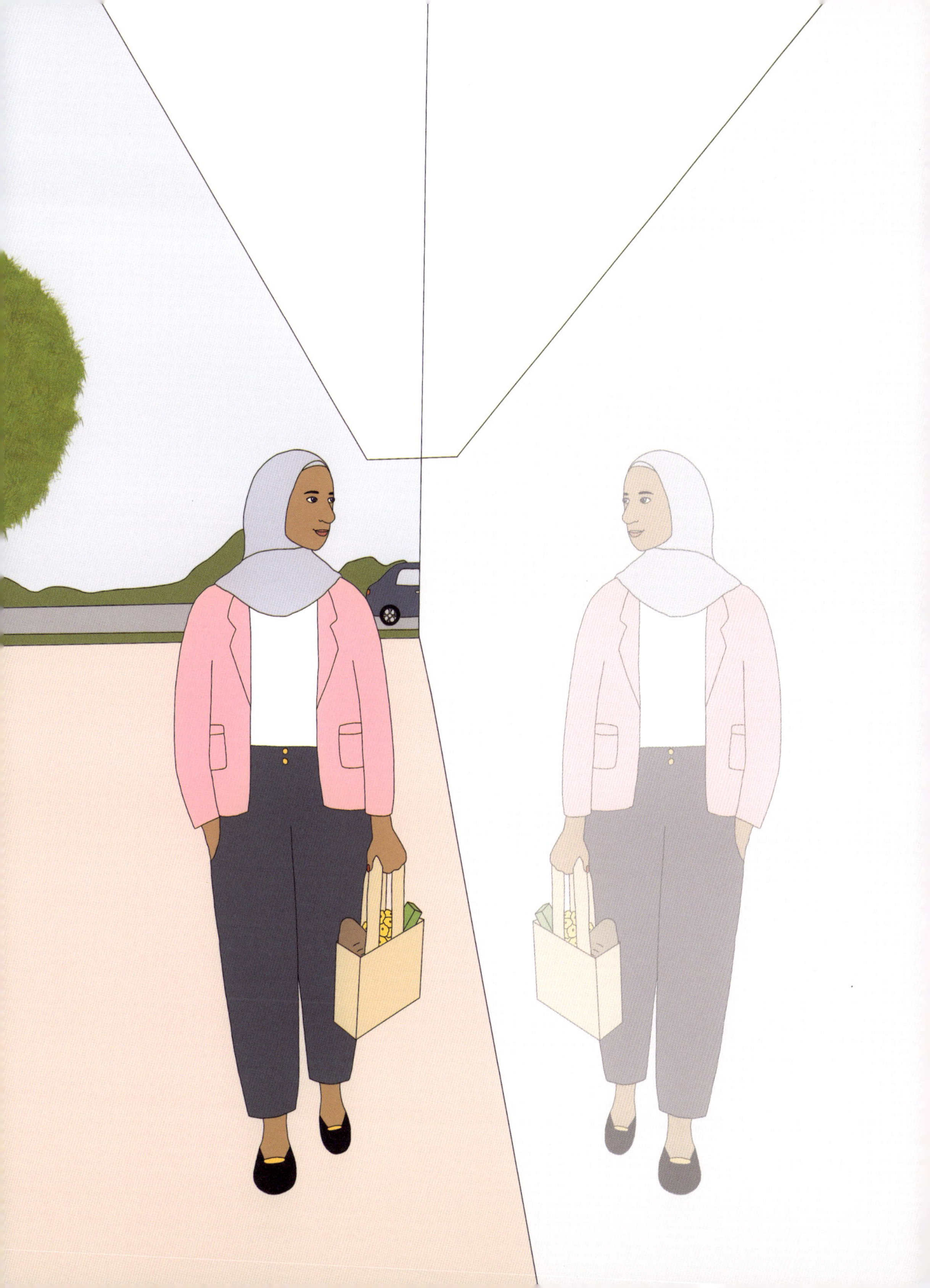

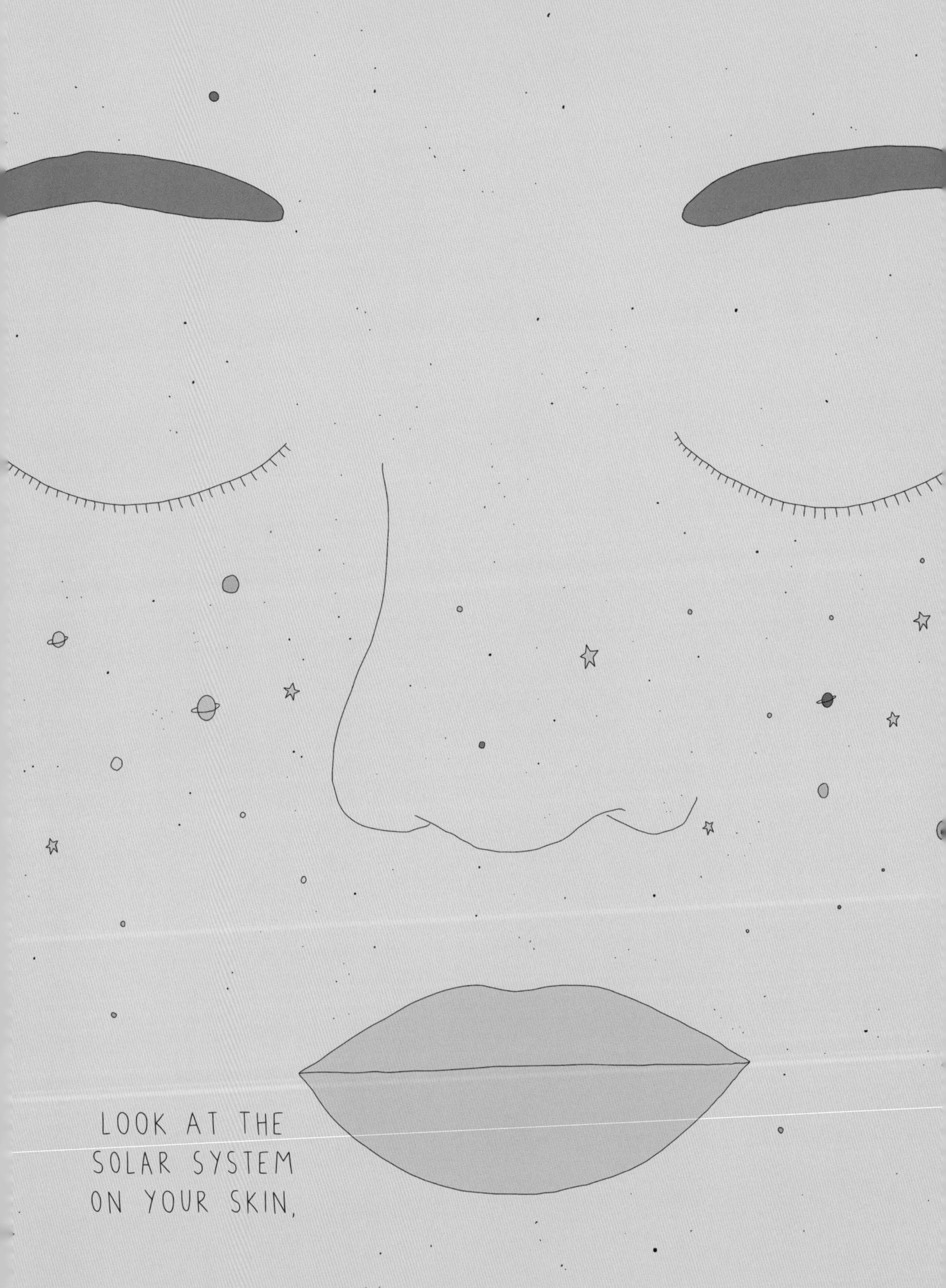
LOOK AT THE
SOLAR SYSTEM
ON YOUR SKIN,

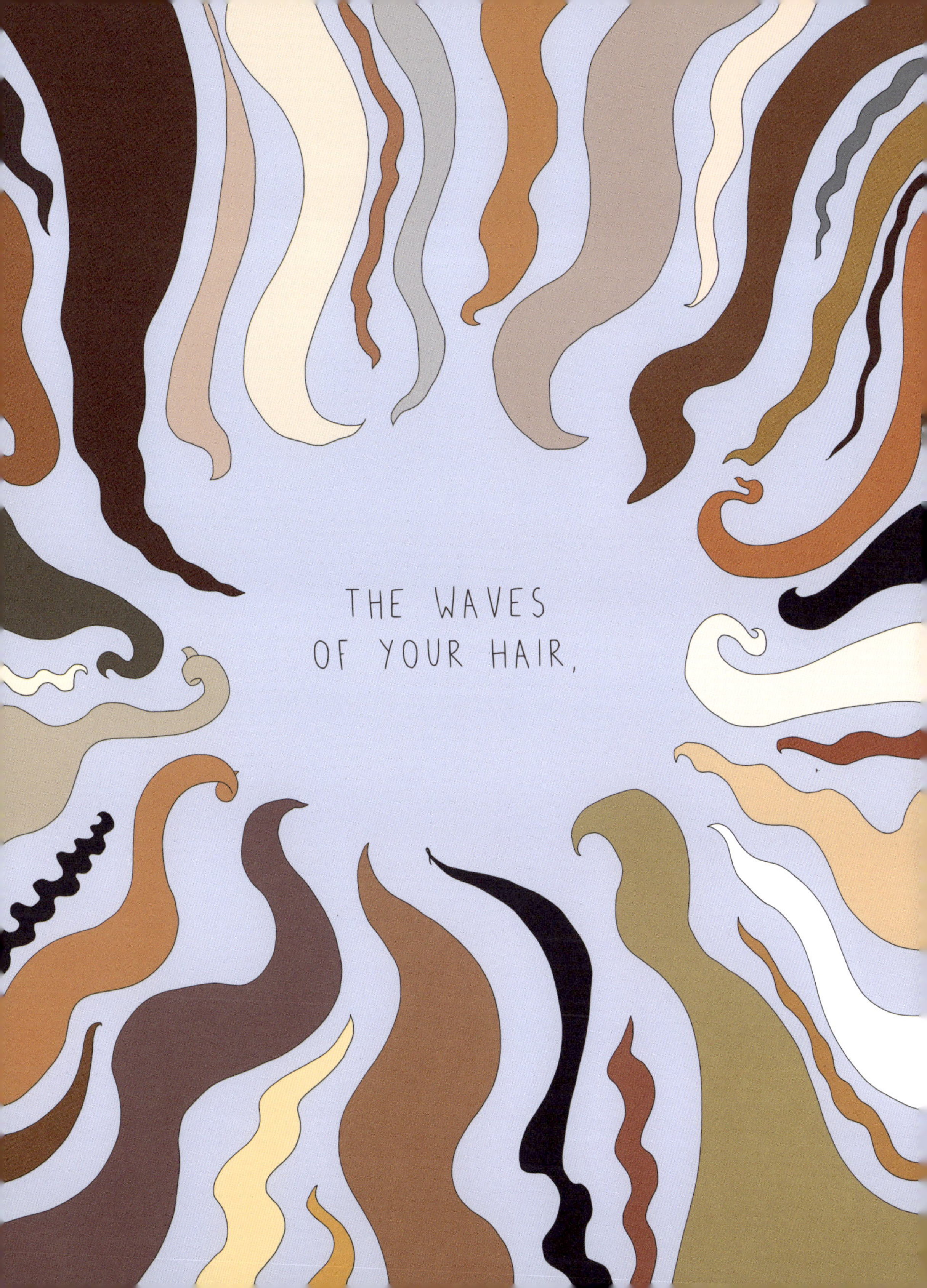
THE WAVES
OF YOUR HAIR,

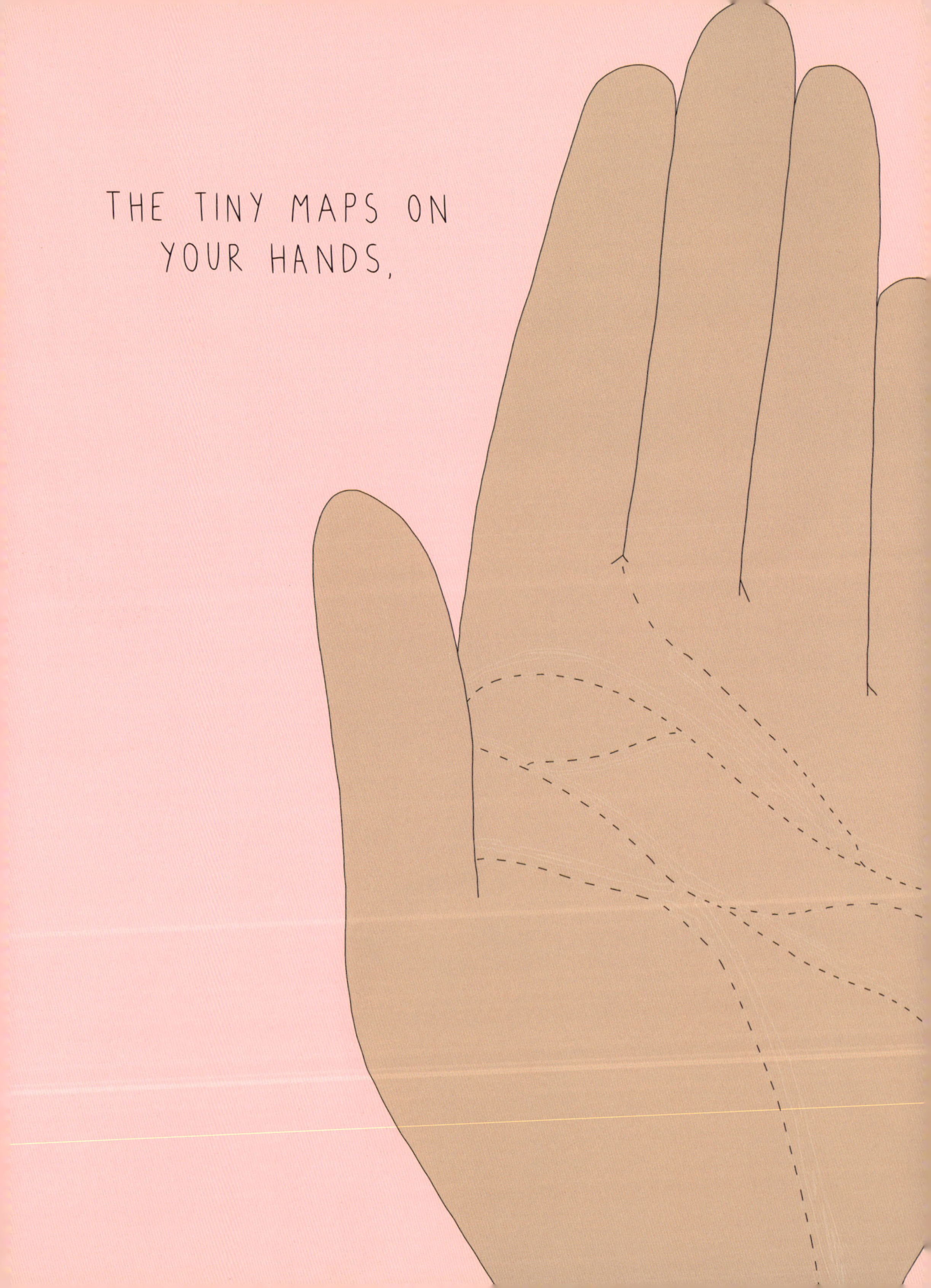
THE TINY MAPS ON
YOUR HANDS,

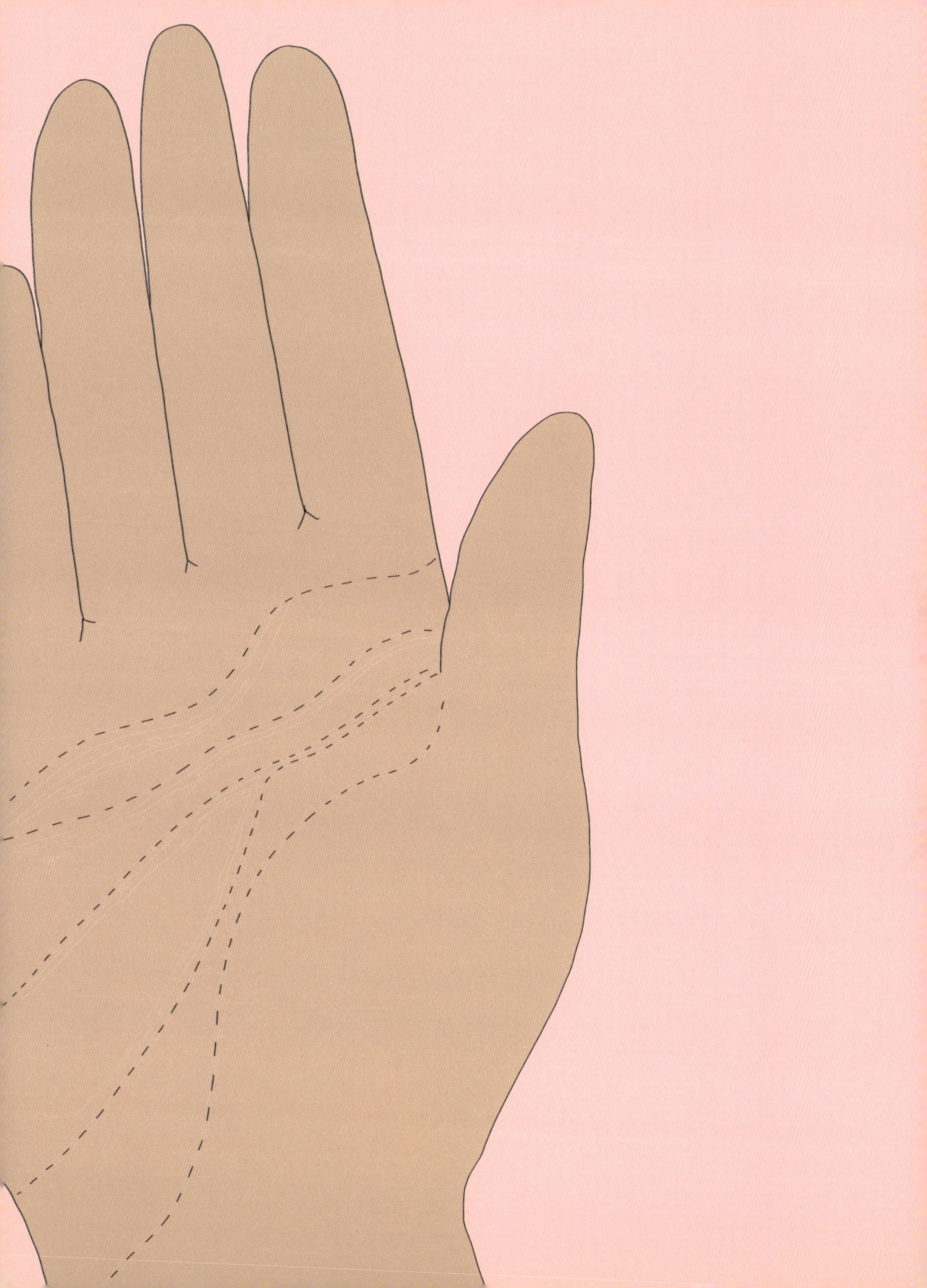

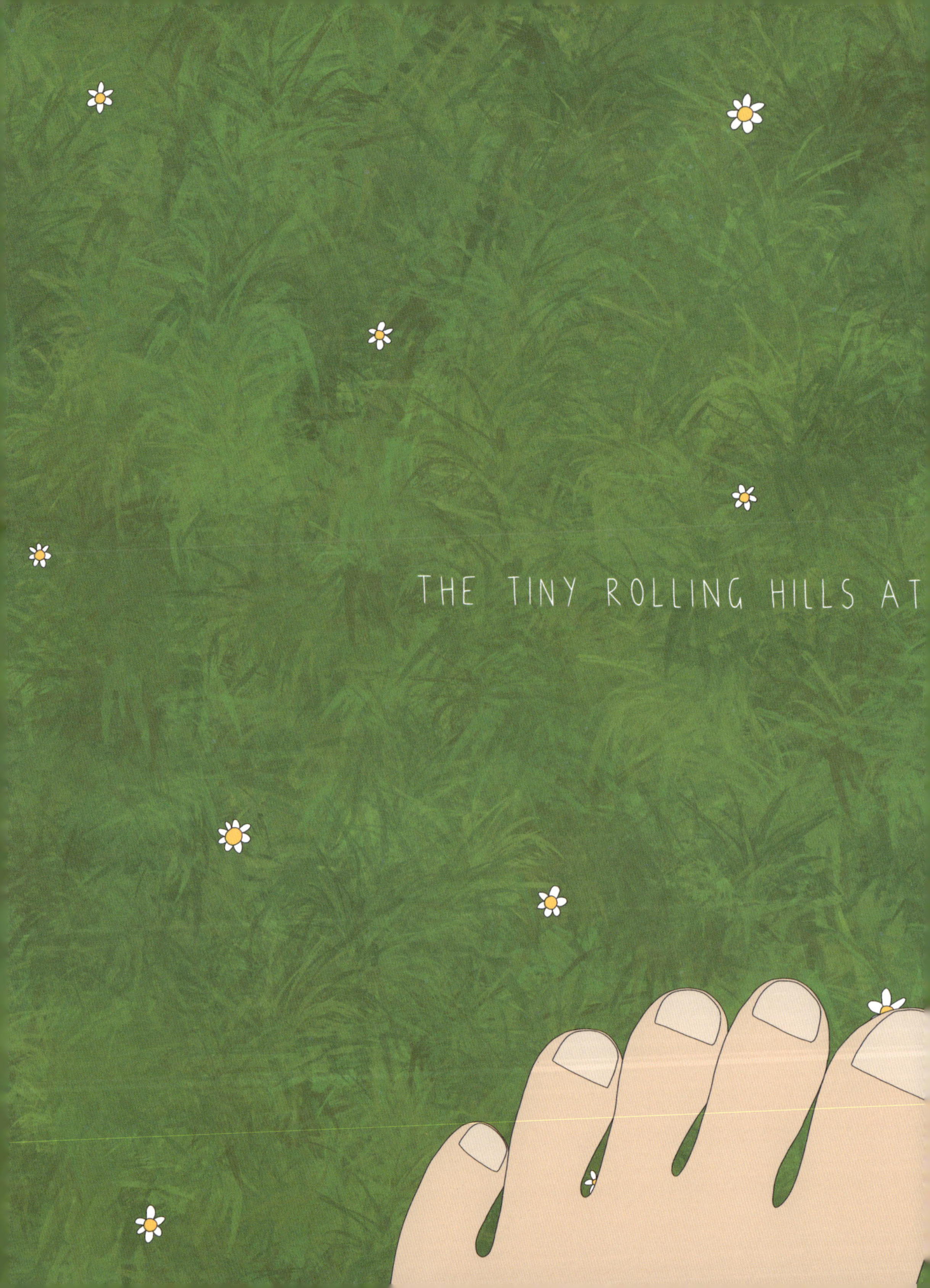
THE TINY ROLLING HILLS AT

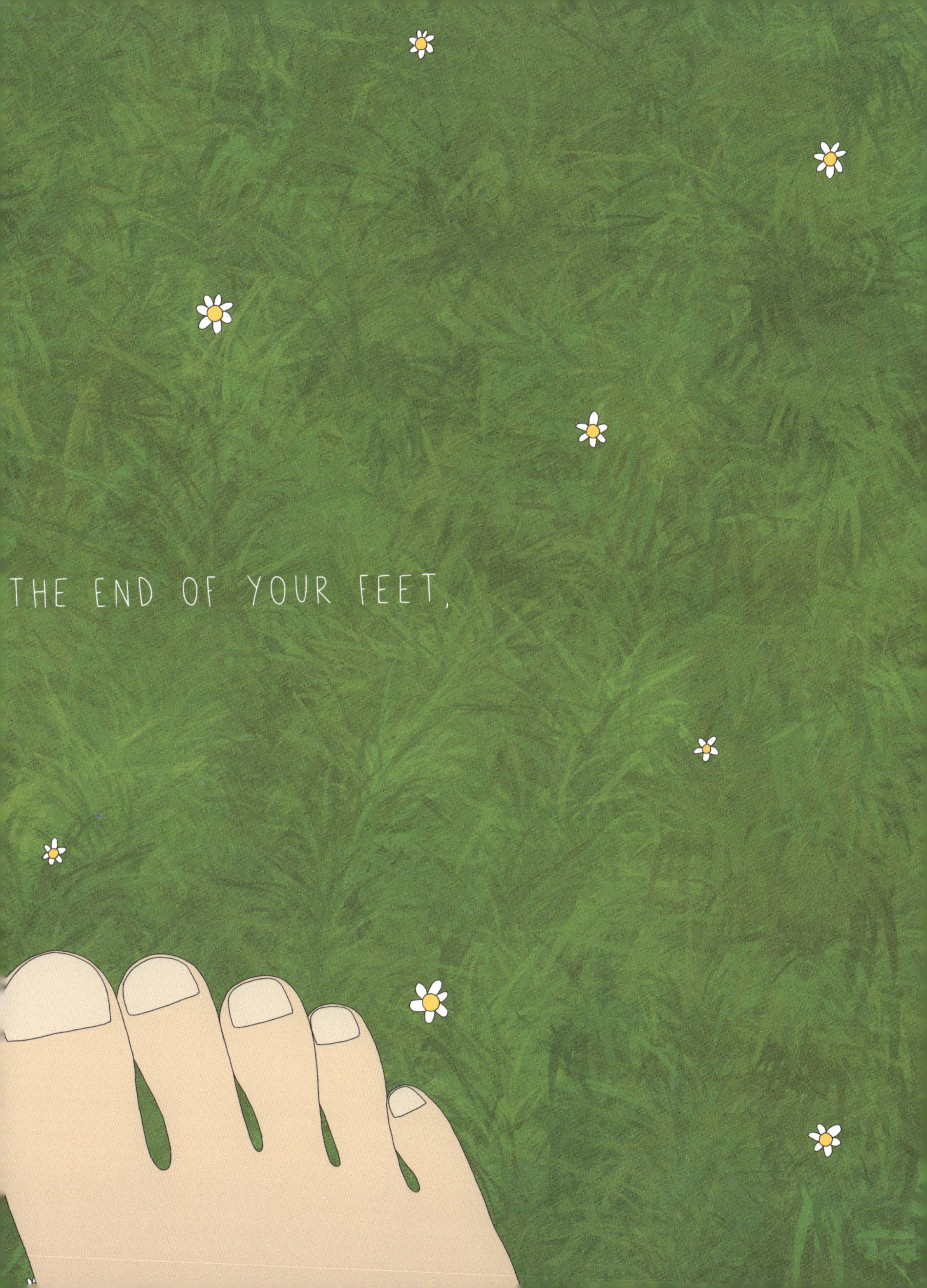
THE END OF YOUR FEET,

THE VALLEYS OF YOUR BELLY,

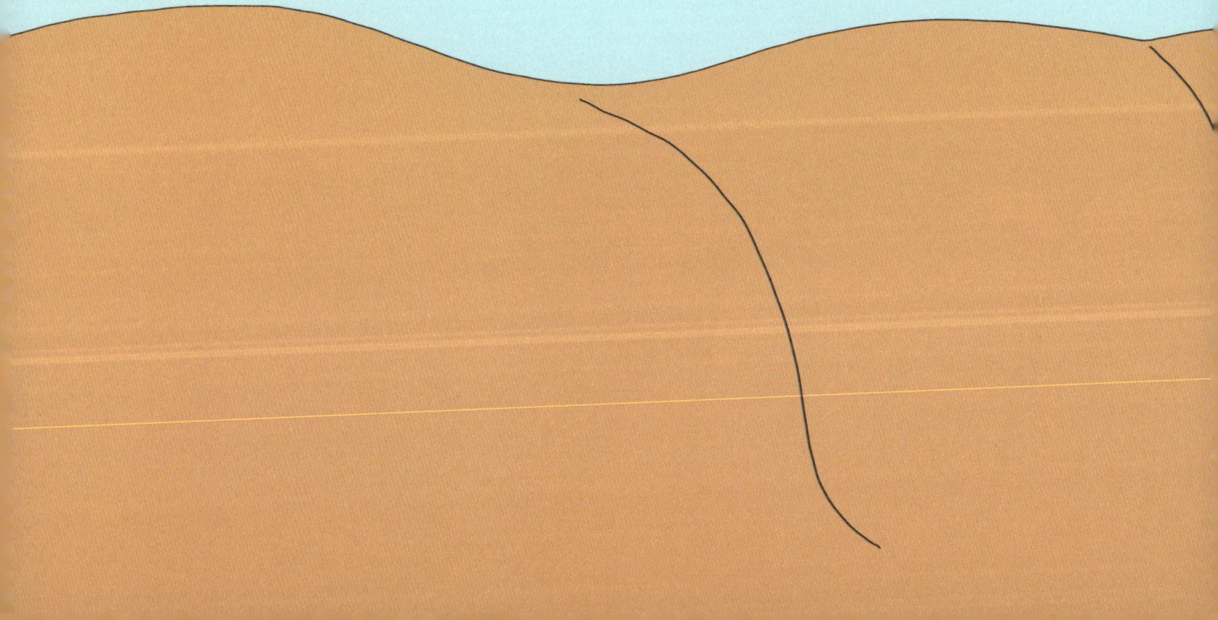

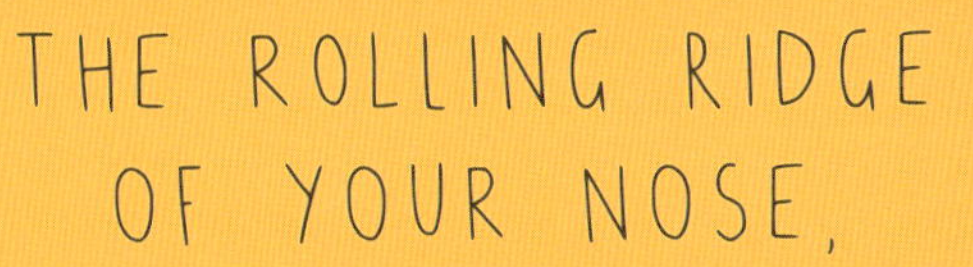
THE ROLLING RIDGE
OF YOUR NOSE,

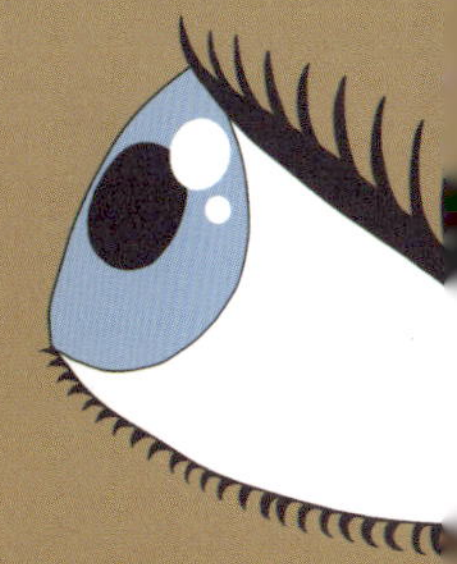

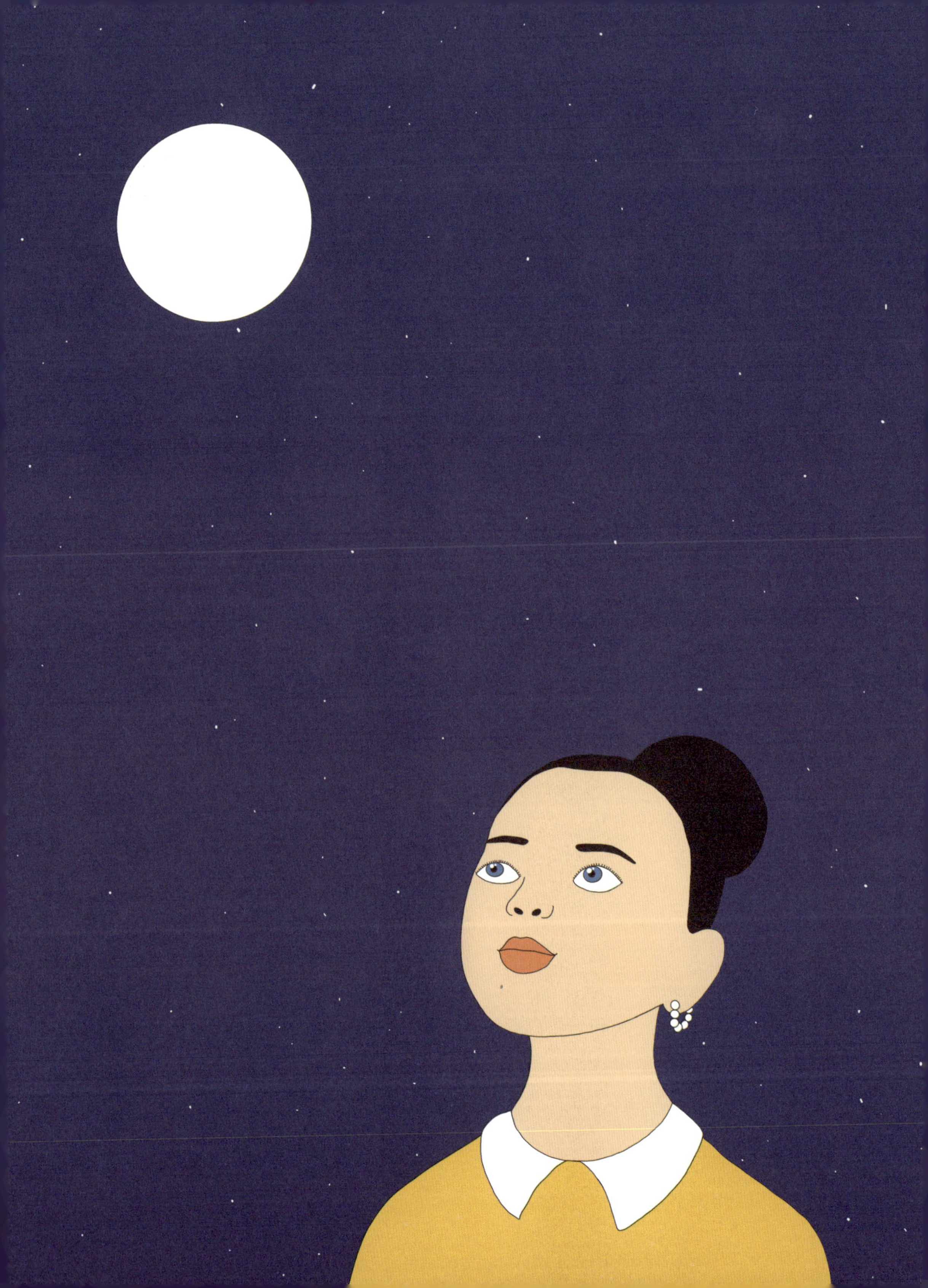

YOUR EYES SHINING BRIGHT LIKE THE MOON,
YOUR SMILE SPARKLING LIKE THE STARS.

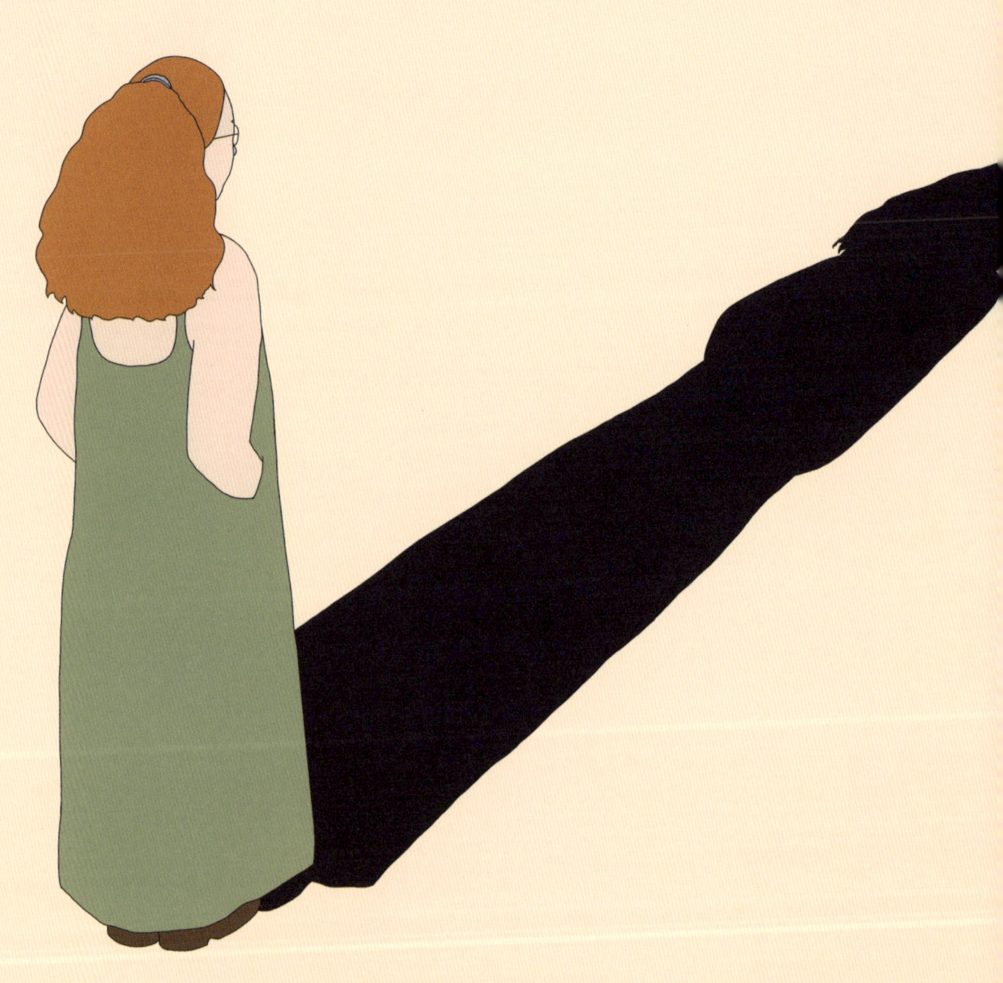

TAKE A MOMENT TO THANK YOUR BODY—TO FORGIVE YOUR BODY.

REMEMBER THE ENORMOUS JOURNEY IT'S BEEN ON, AND KNOW IT'S DOING THE BEST IT CAN FOR YOU EVERY SINGLE DAY.

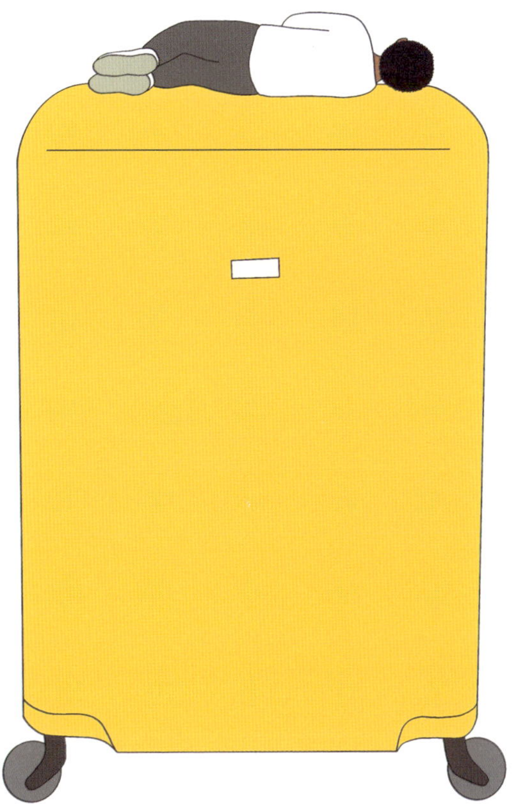

KEEP LEARNING HOW TO
SHOW YOUR BODY LOVE.

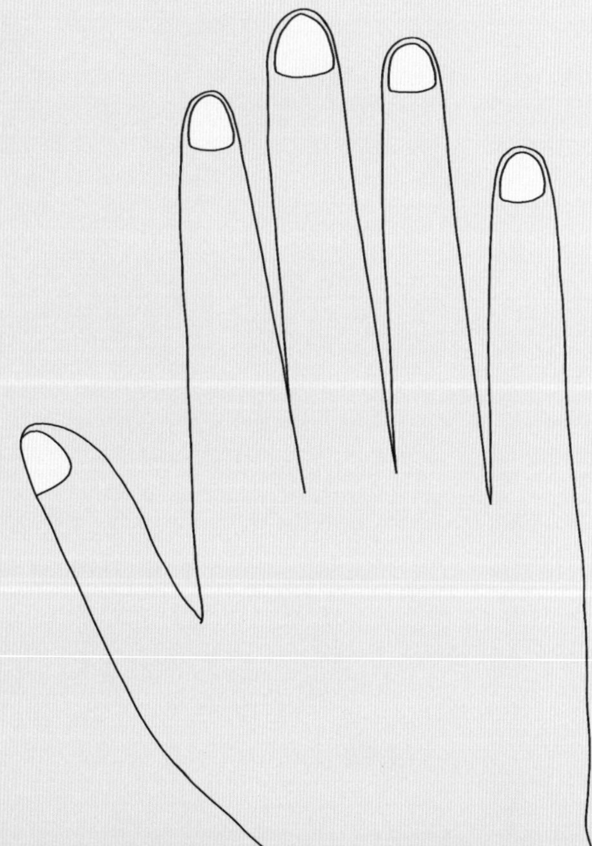

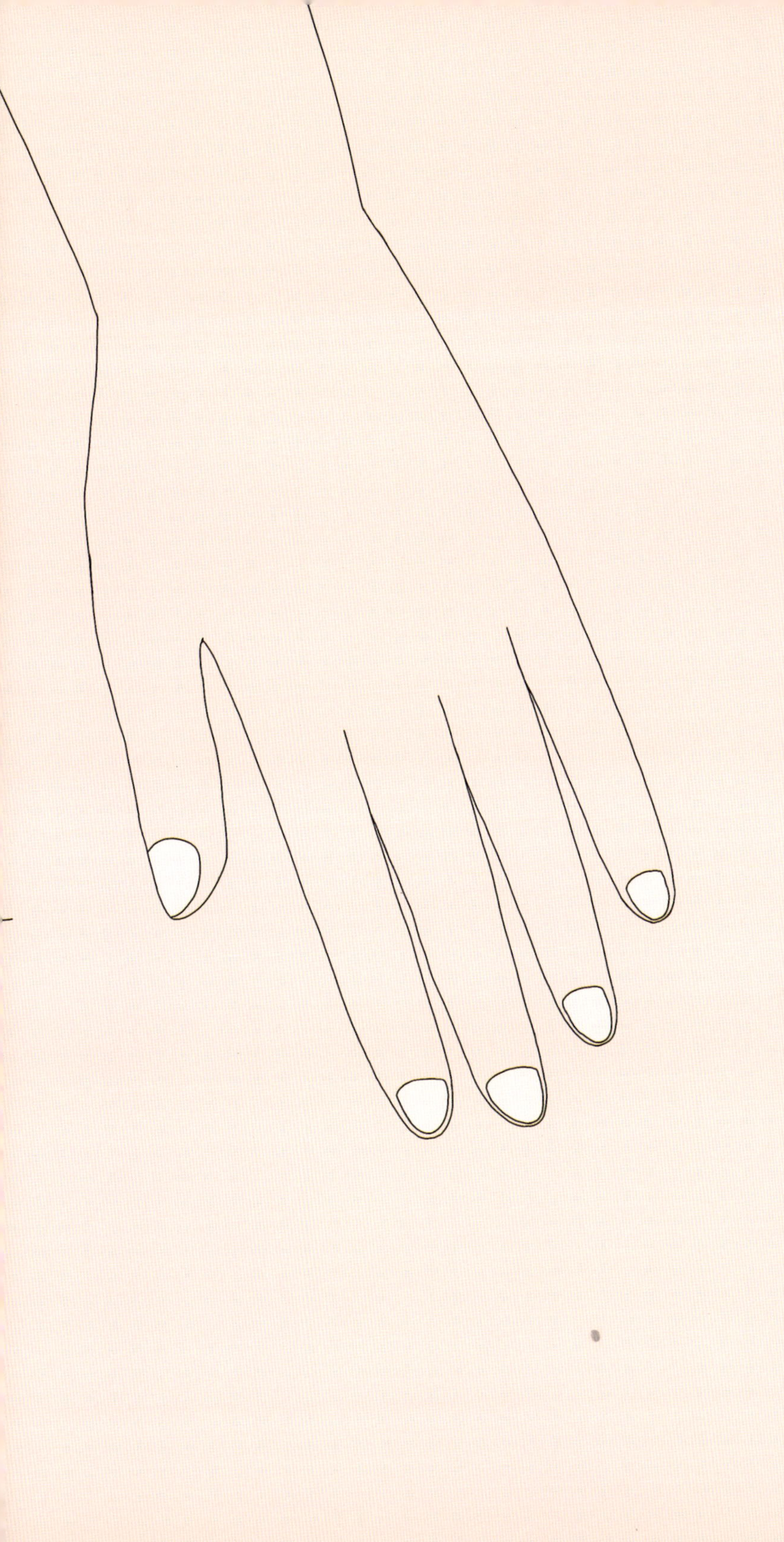

YOU MIGHT WANT TO
SHOUT THE LOVE YOU
FEEL FOR YOURSELF
FROM THE ROOFTOPS,

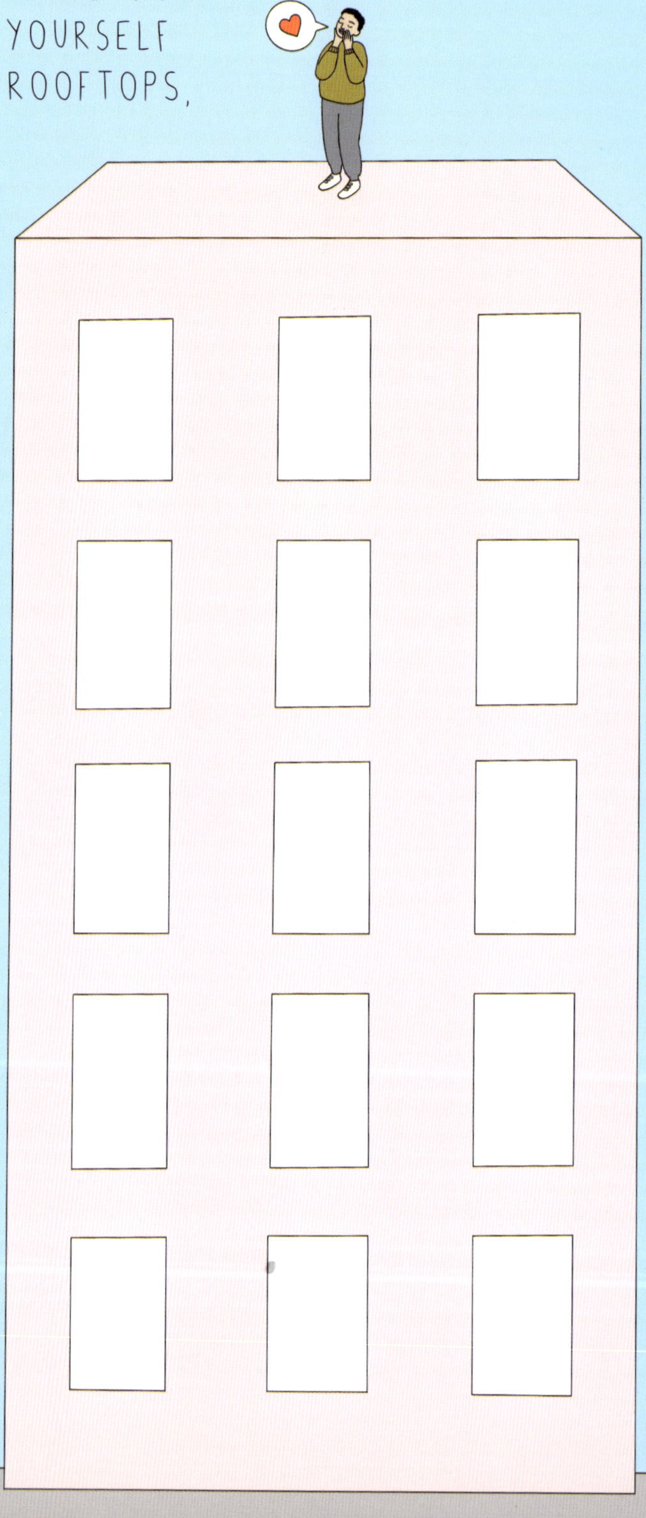

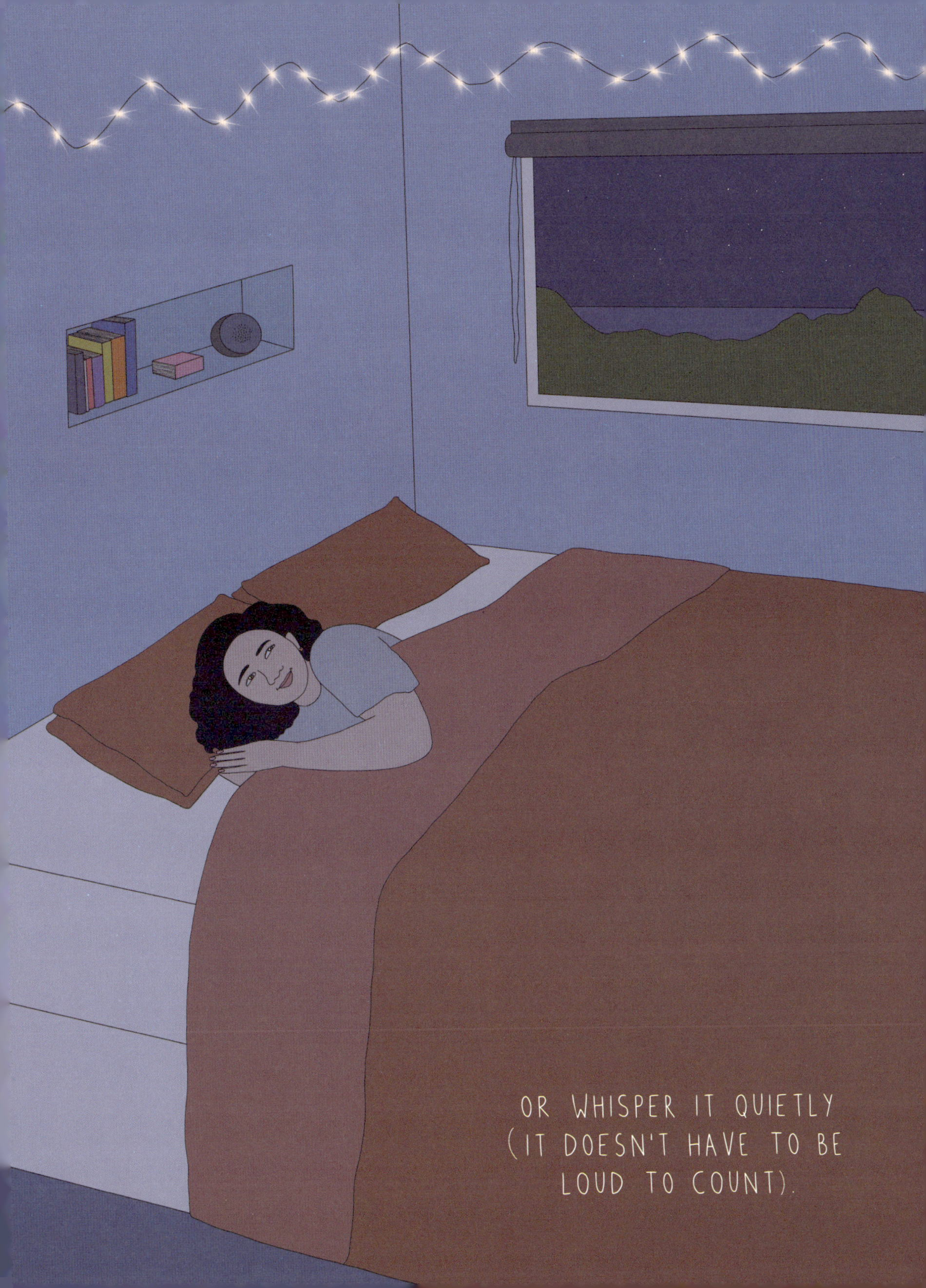
OR WHISPER IT QUIETLY
(IT DOESN'T HAVE TO BE
LOUD TO COUNT).

LET IT CONTINUE TO BE A PLACE OF WONDER.

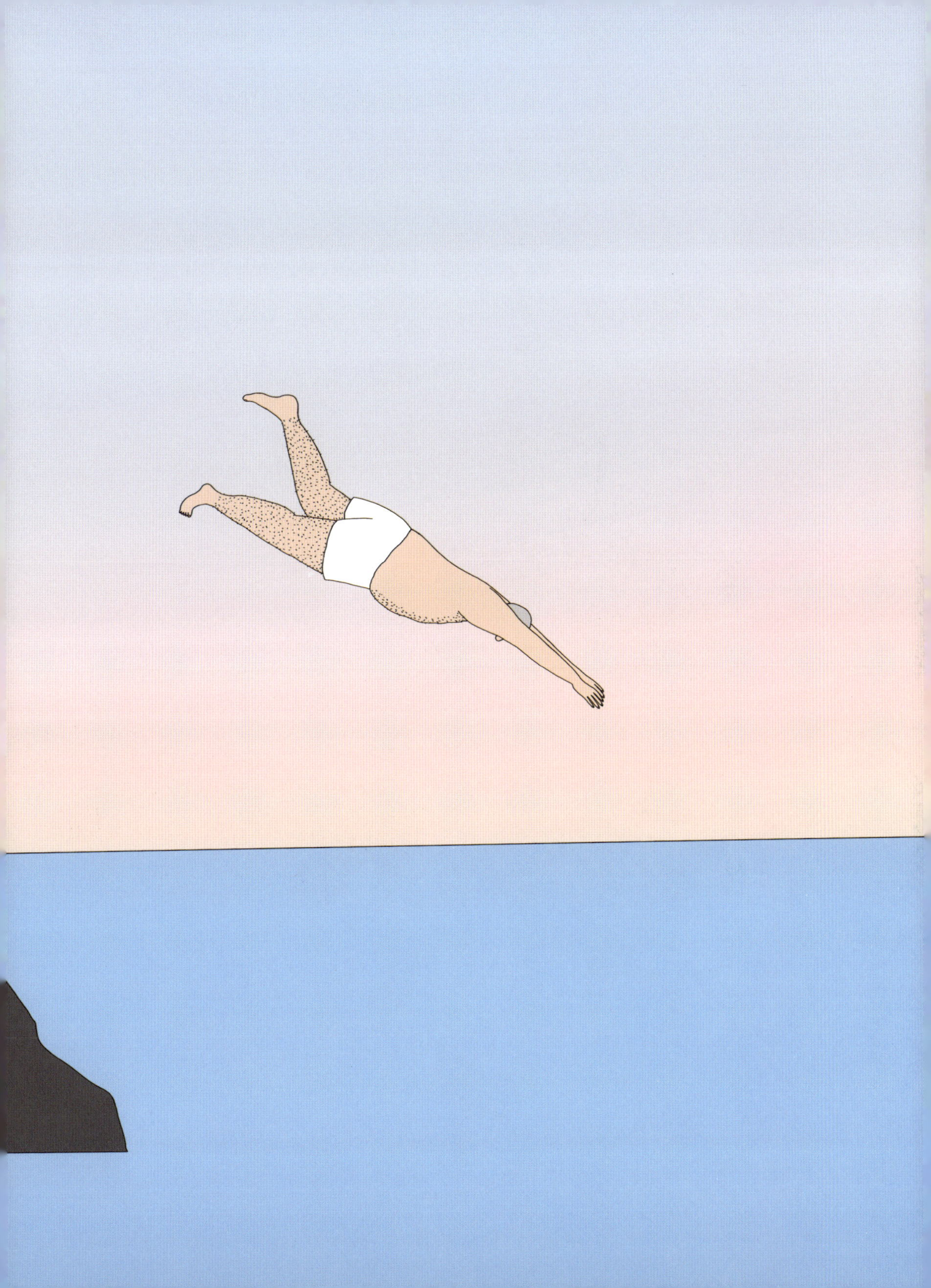

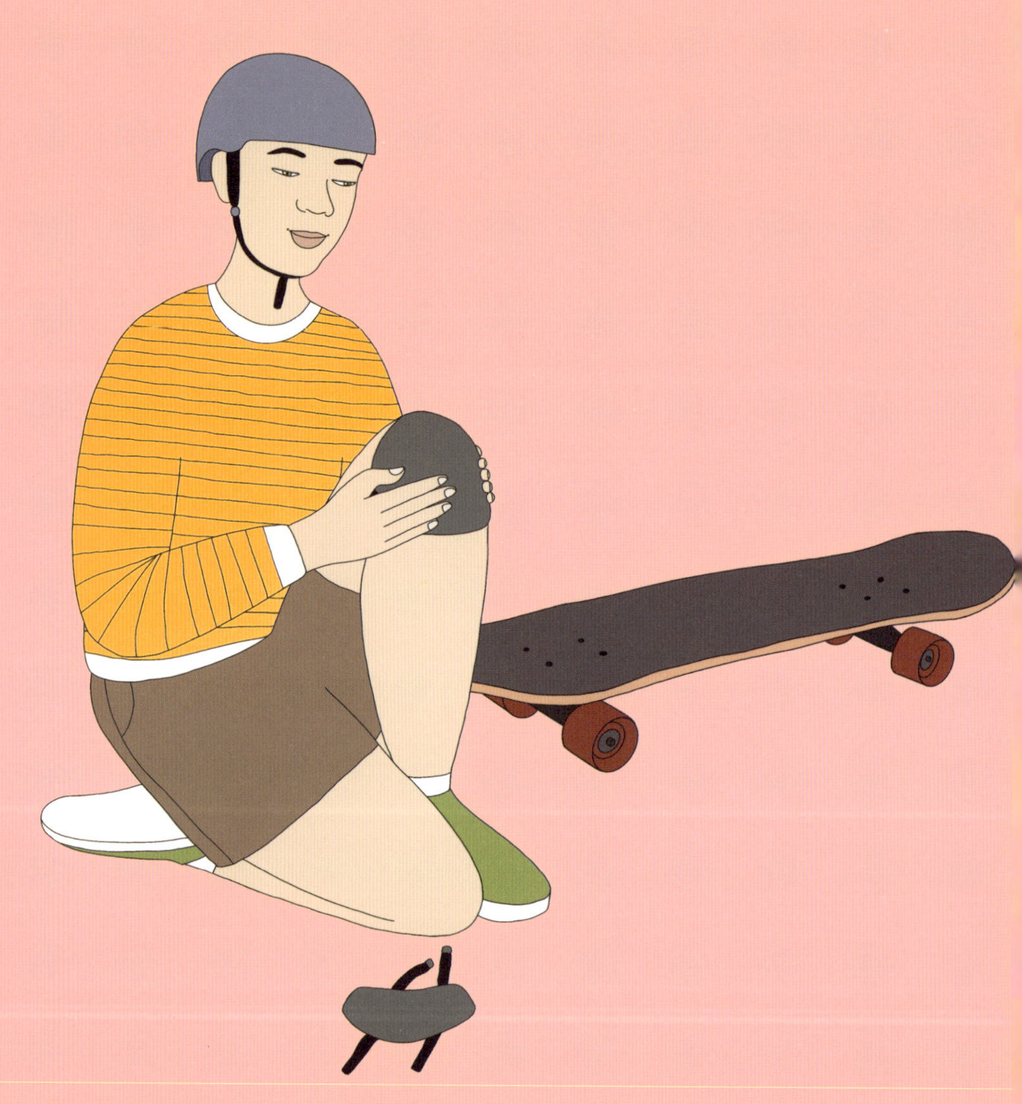

PROTECT IT.

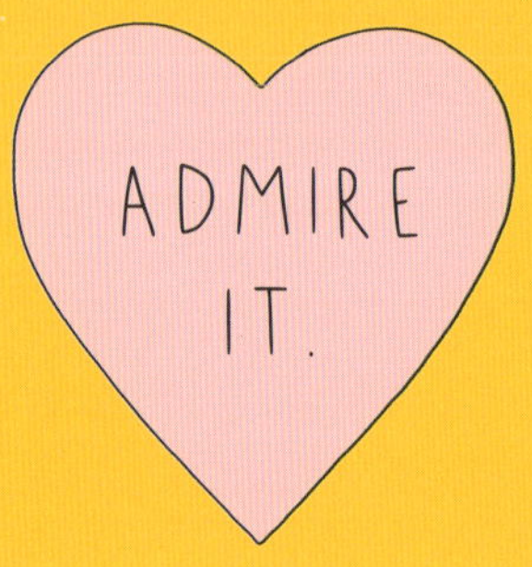
ADMIRE
IT.

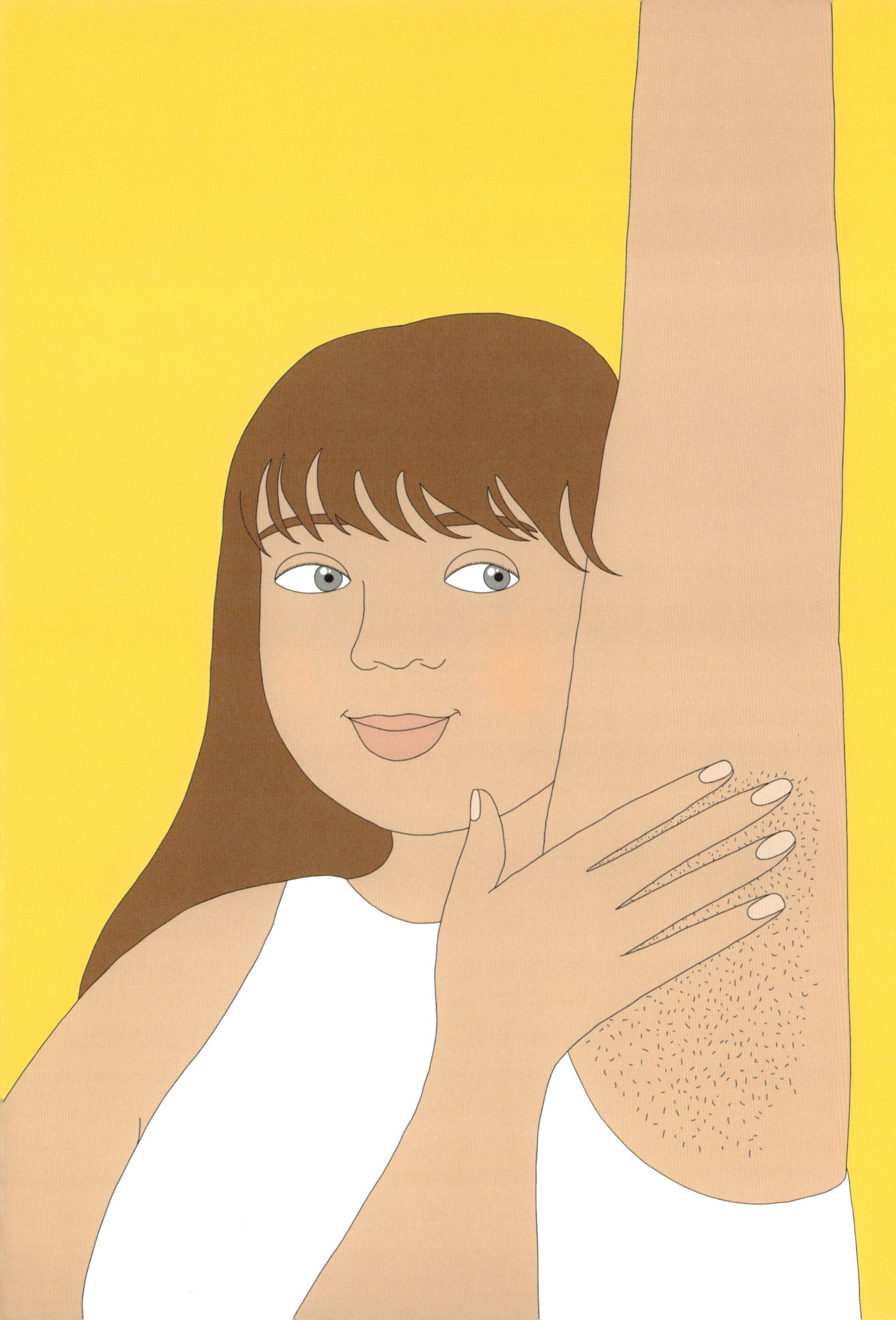

CELEBRATE IT.

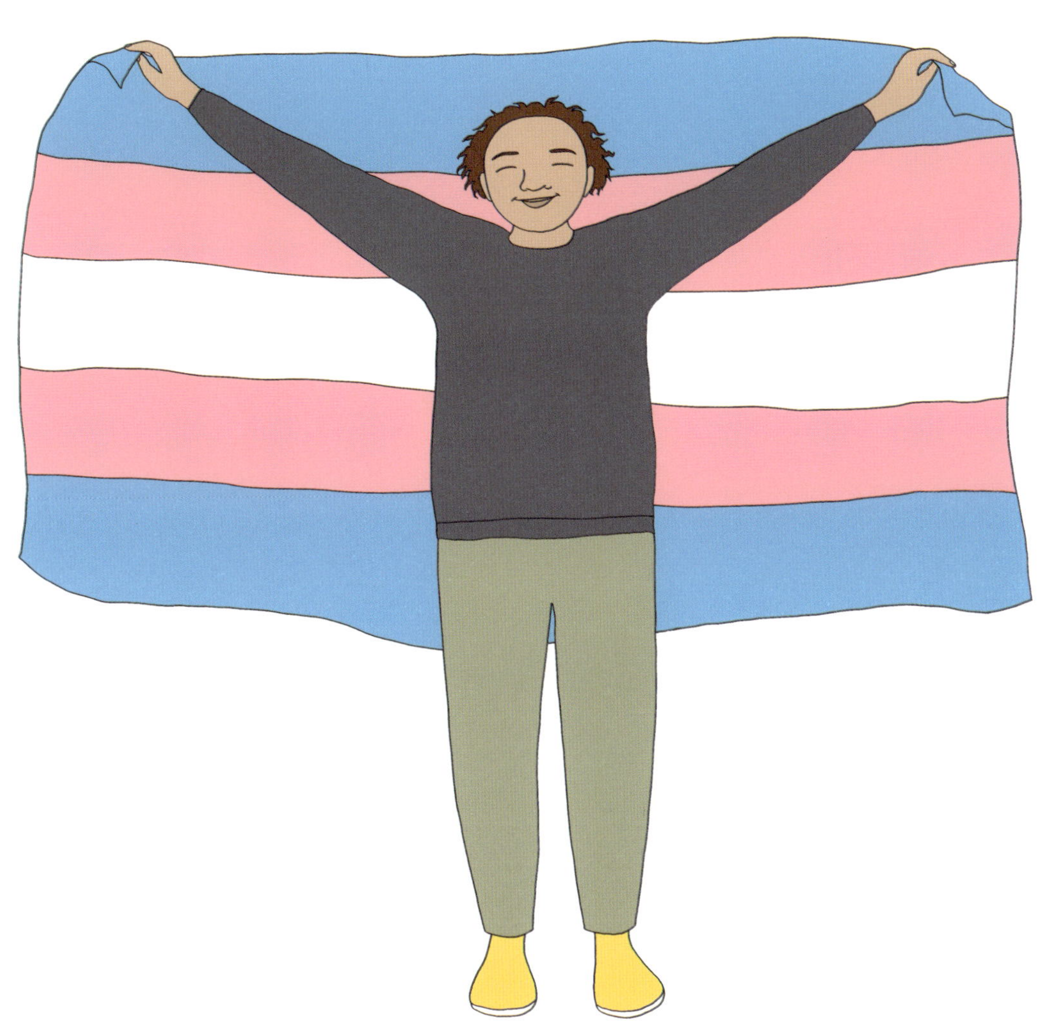

RECLAIM THE MAGIC.

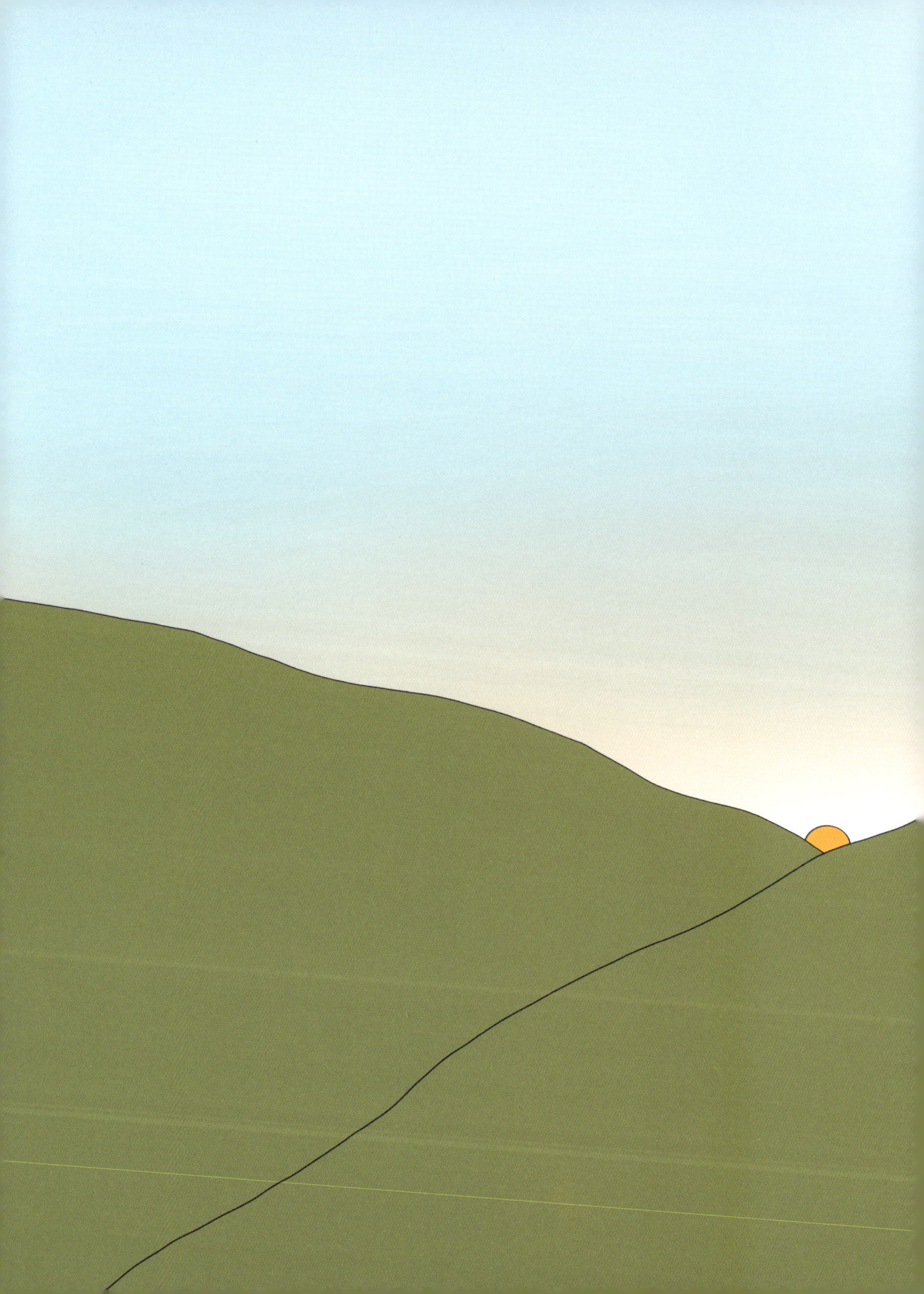

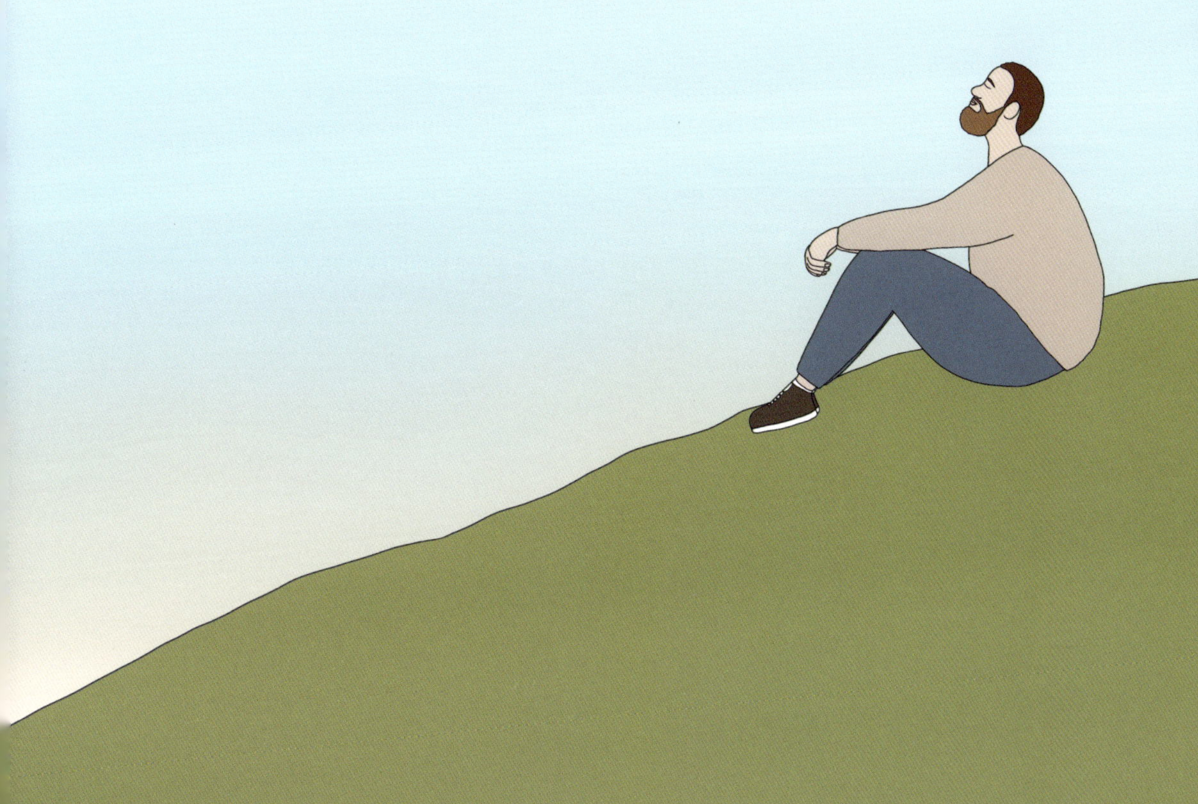

FEEL YOUR LUNGS FILL WITH THE FRESH MORNING AIR.

YOUR HEART POUNDING AS YOU DANCE.

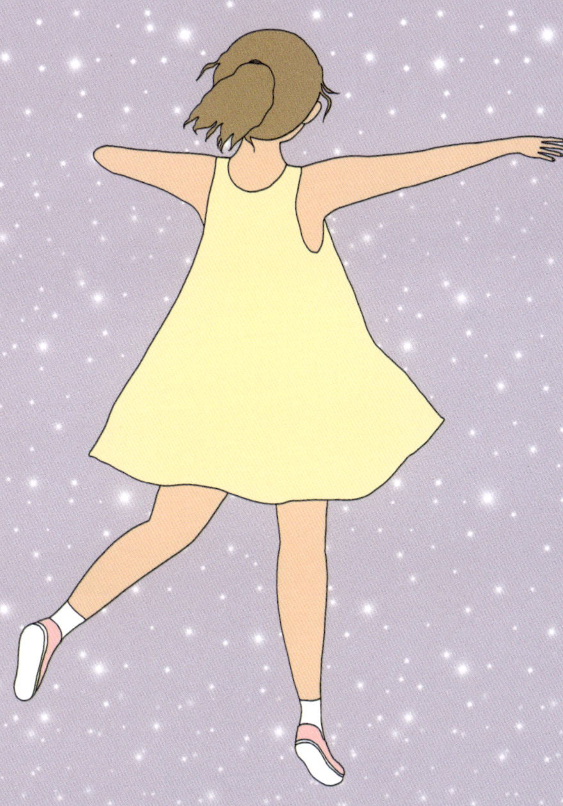

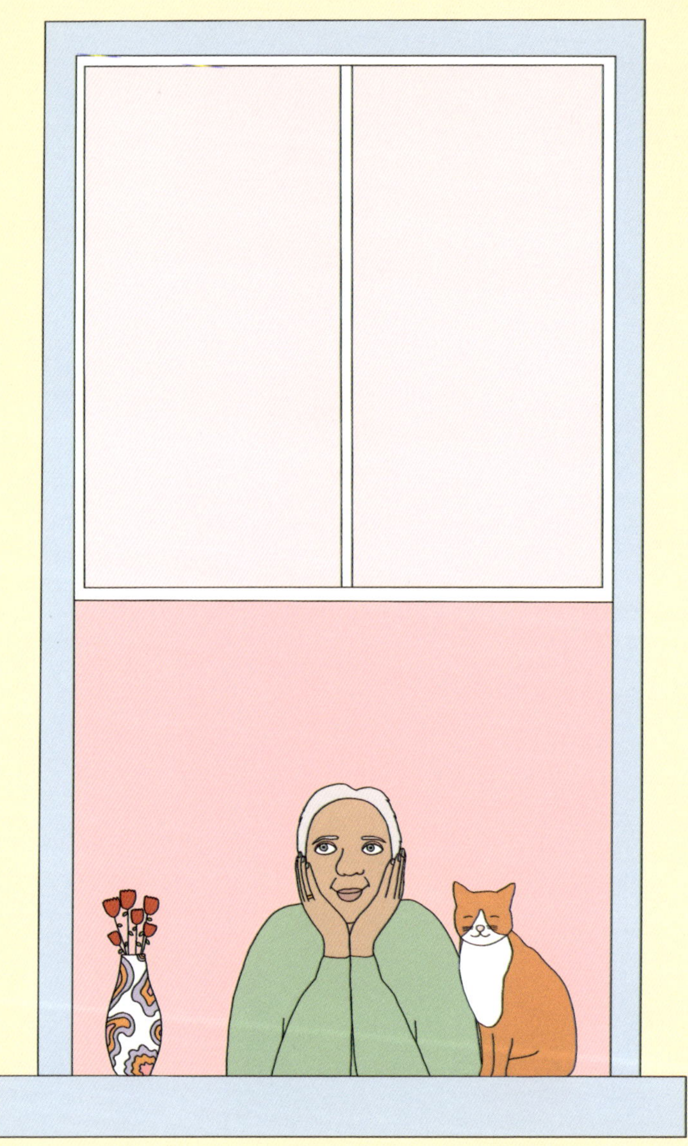

TREASURE EVERY ADVENTURE
YOUR BODY TAKES YOU ON.

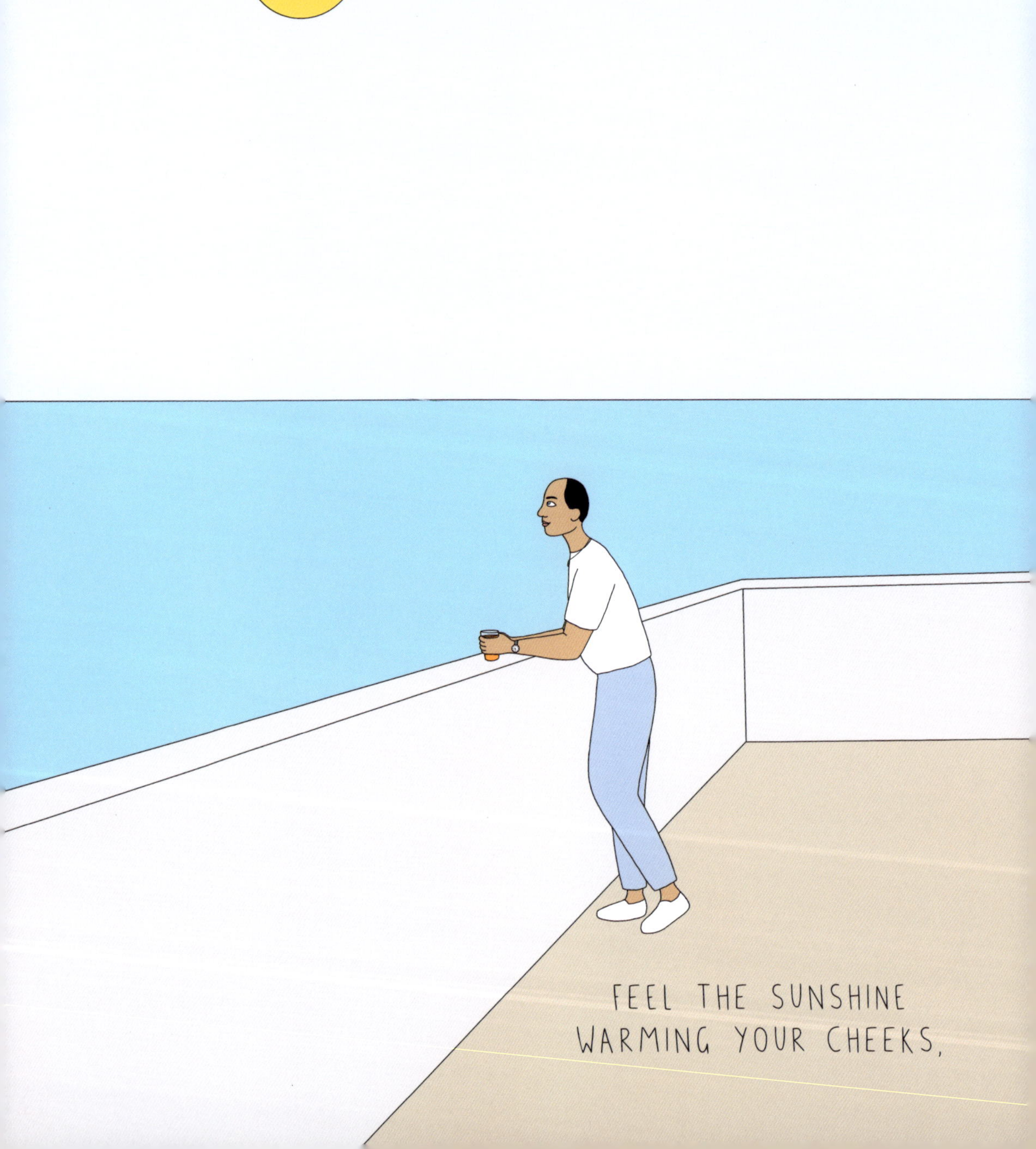
FEEL THE SUNSHINE
WARMING YOUR CHEEKS,

SEE THE OCEAN MEETING YOUR FEET,

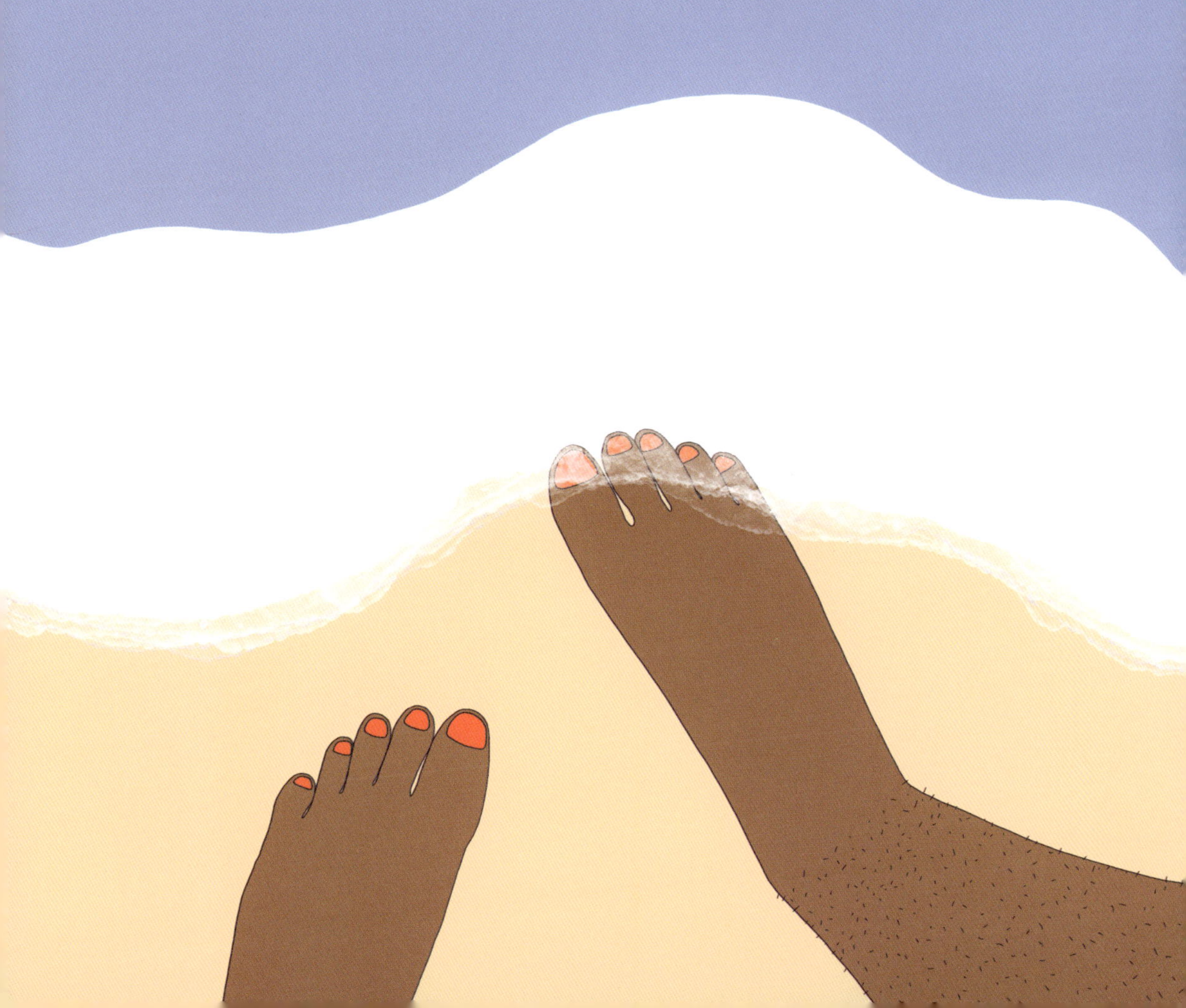

LISTEN TO THE BIRDS
SINGING THEIR MORNING
SONGS FOR YOU.

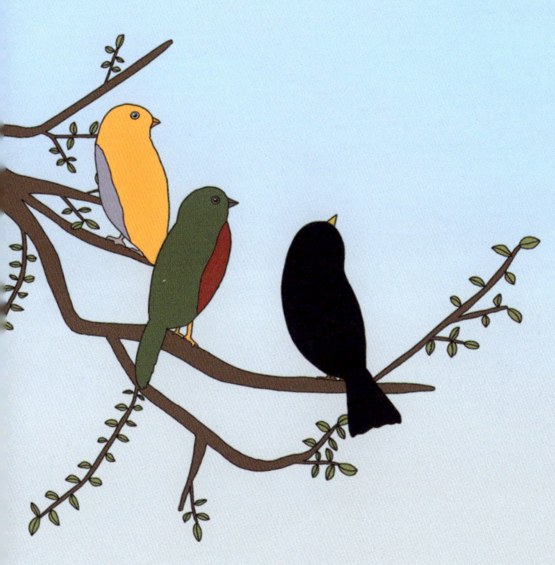
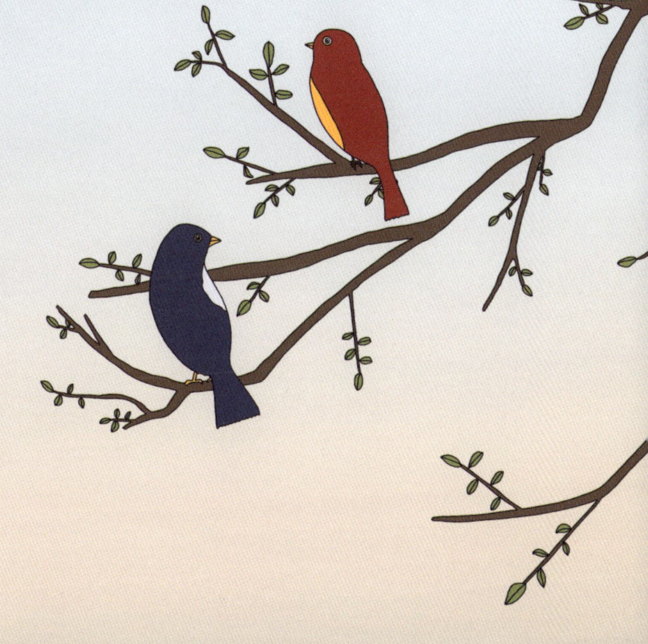

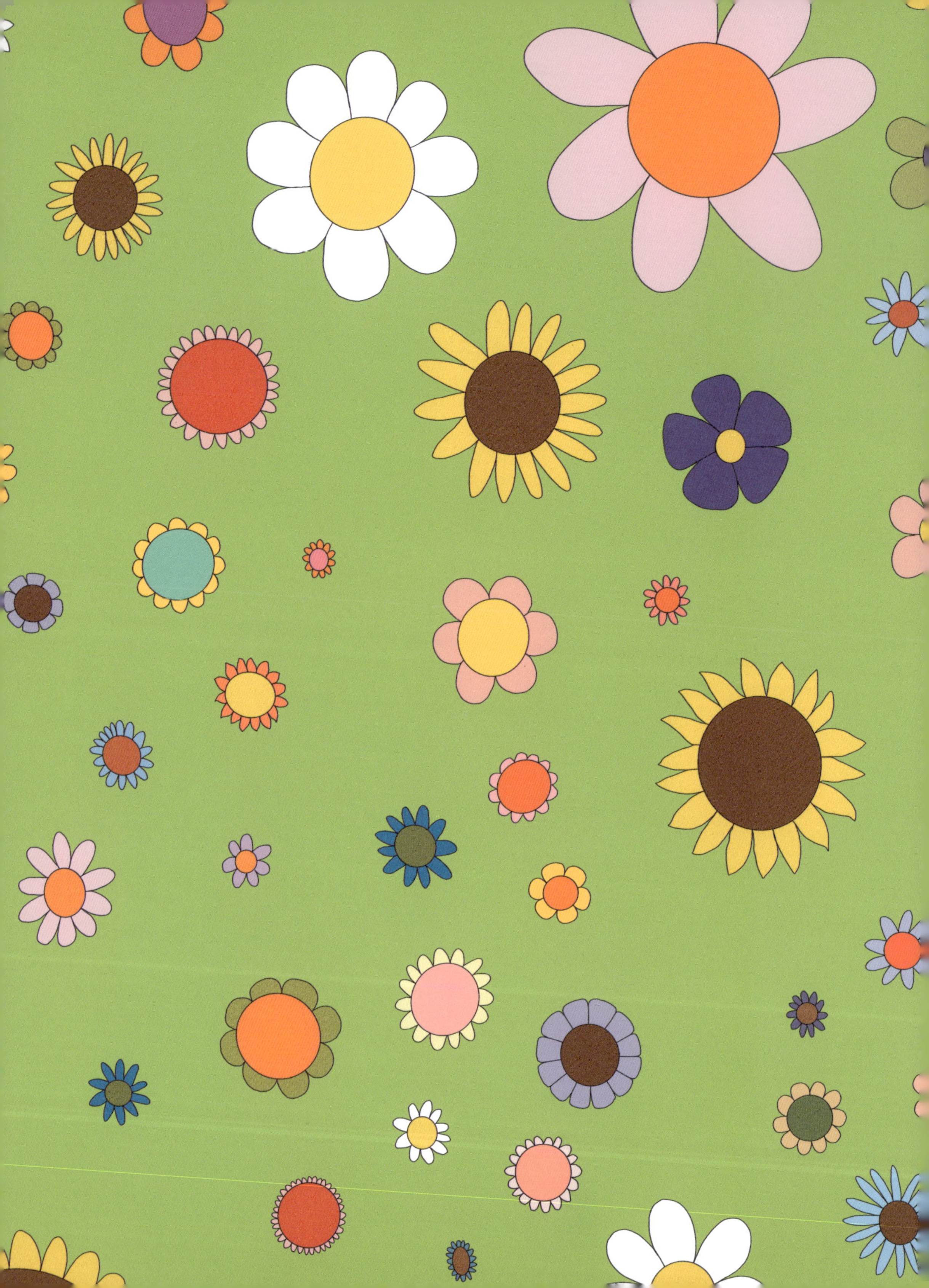

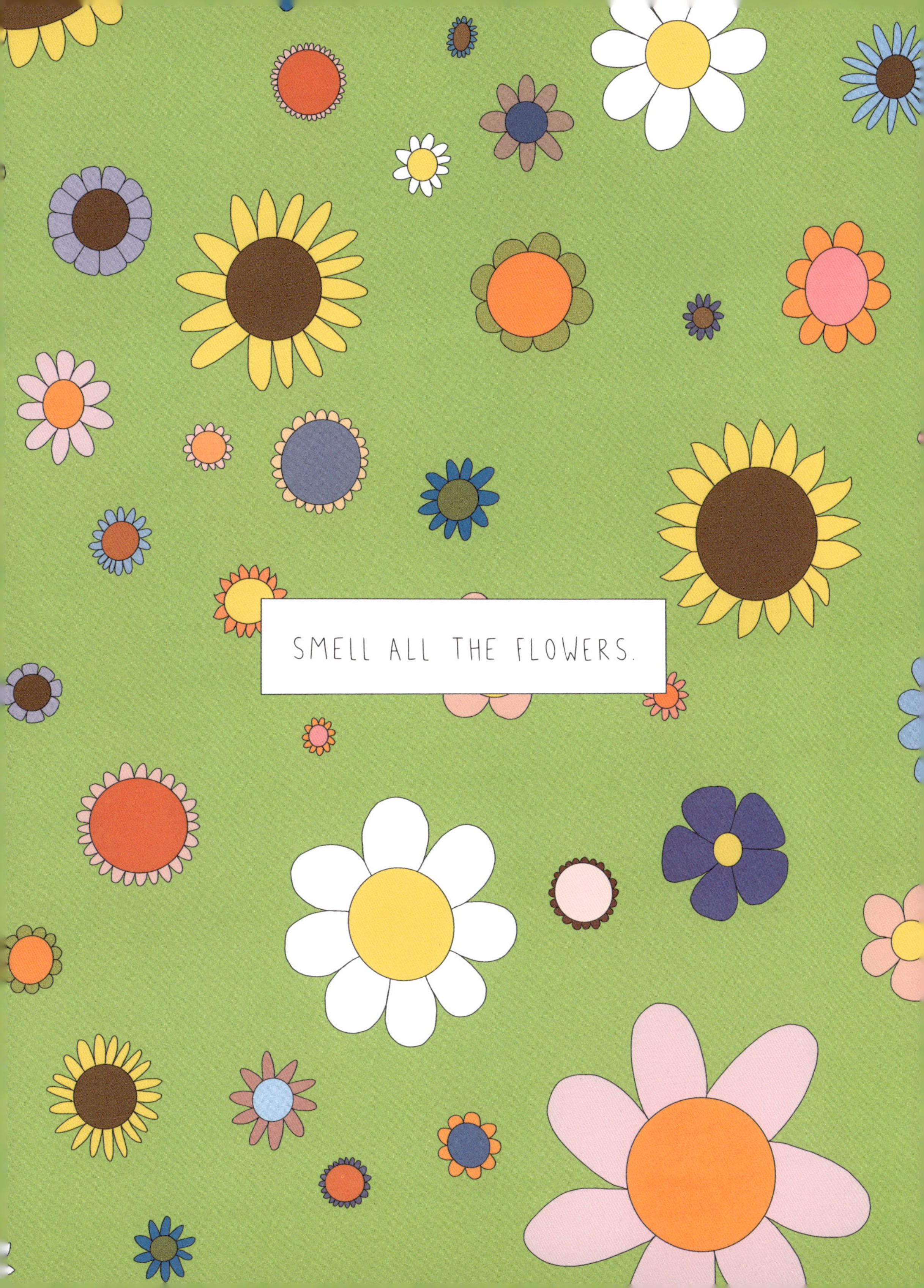
SMELL ALL THE FLOWERS.

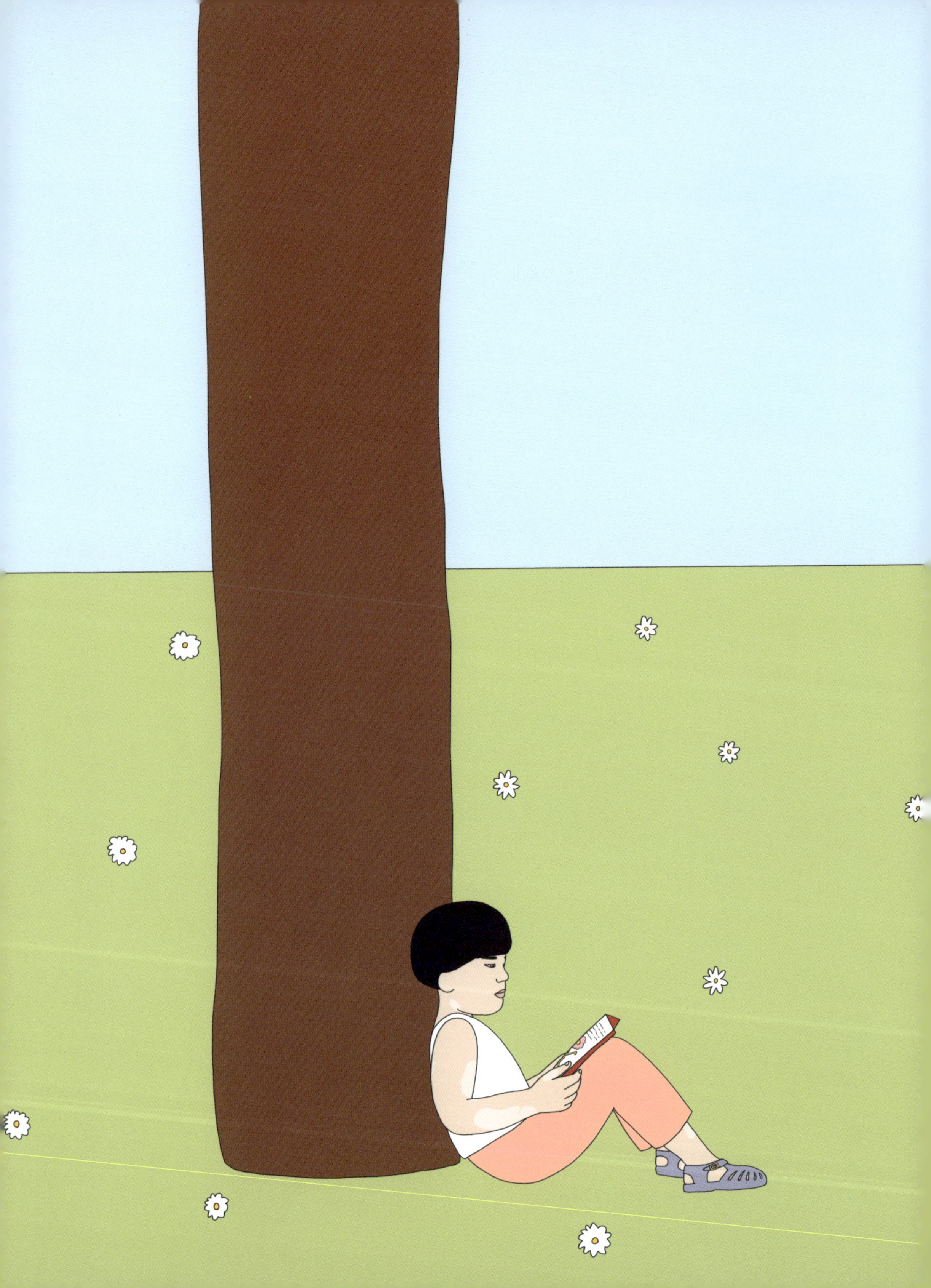

HOLD ON TO THE BEAUTY, THE JOY, THE GIFT...

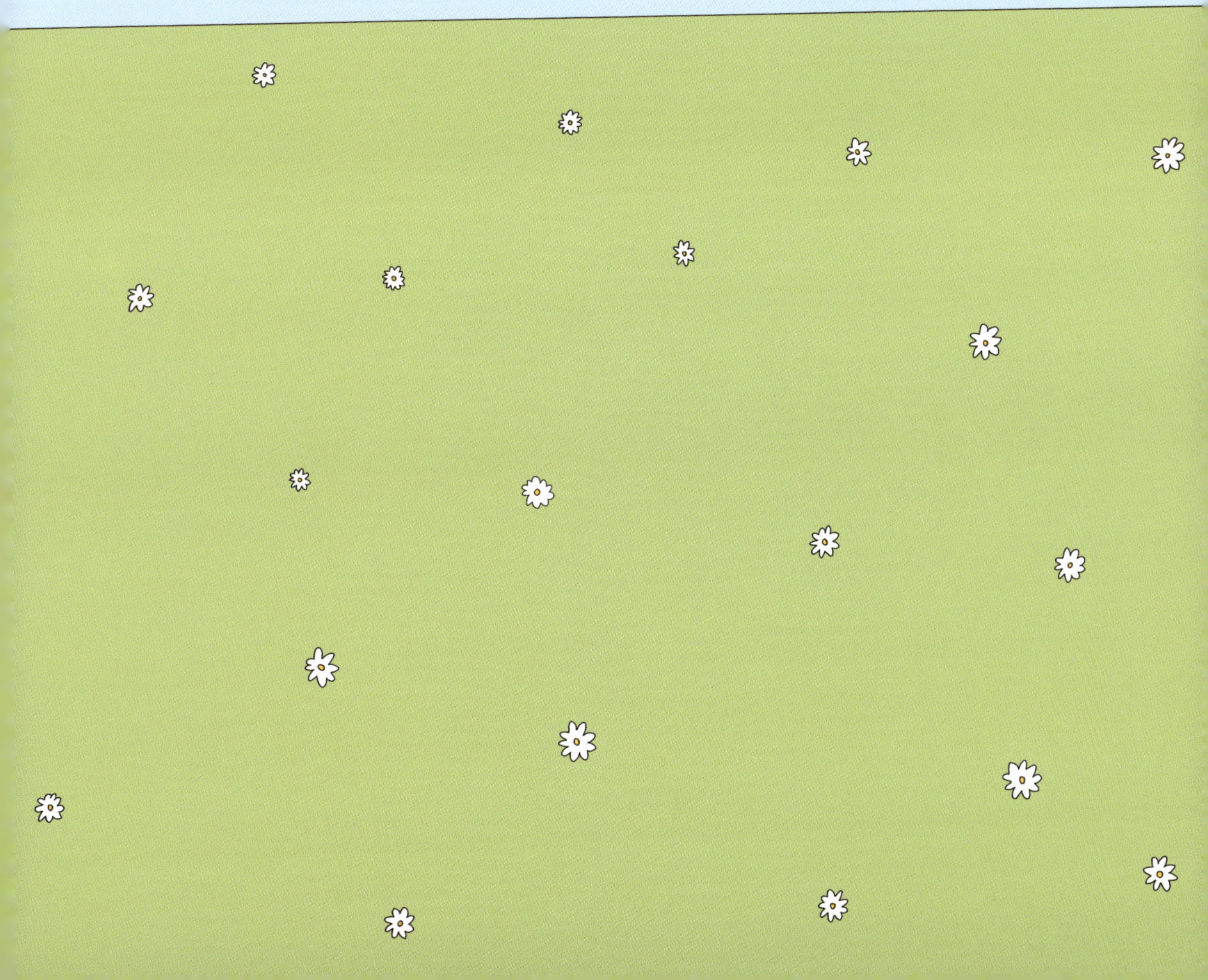

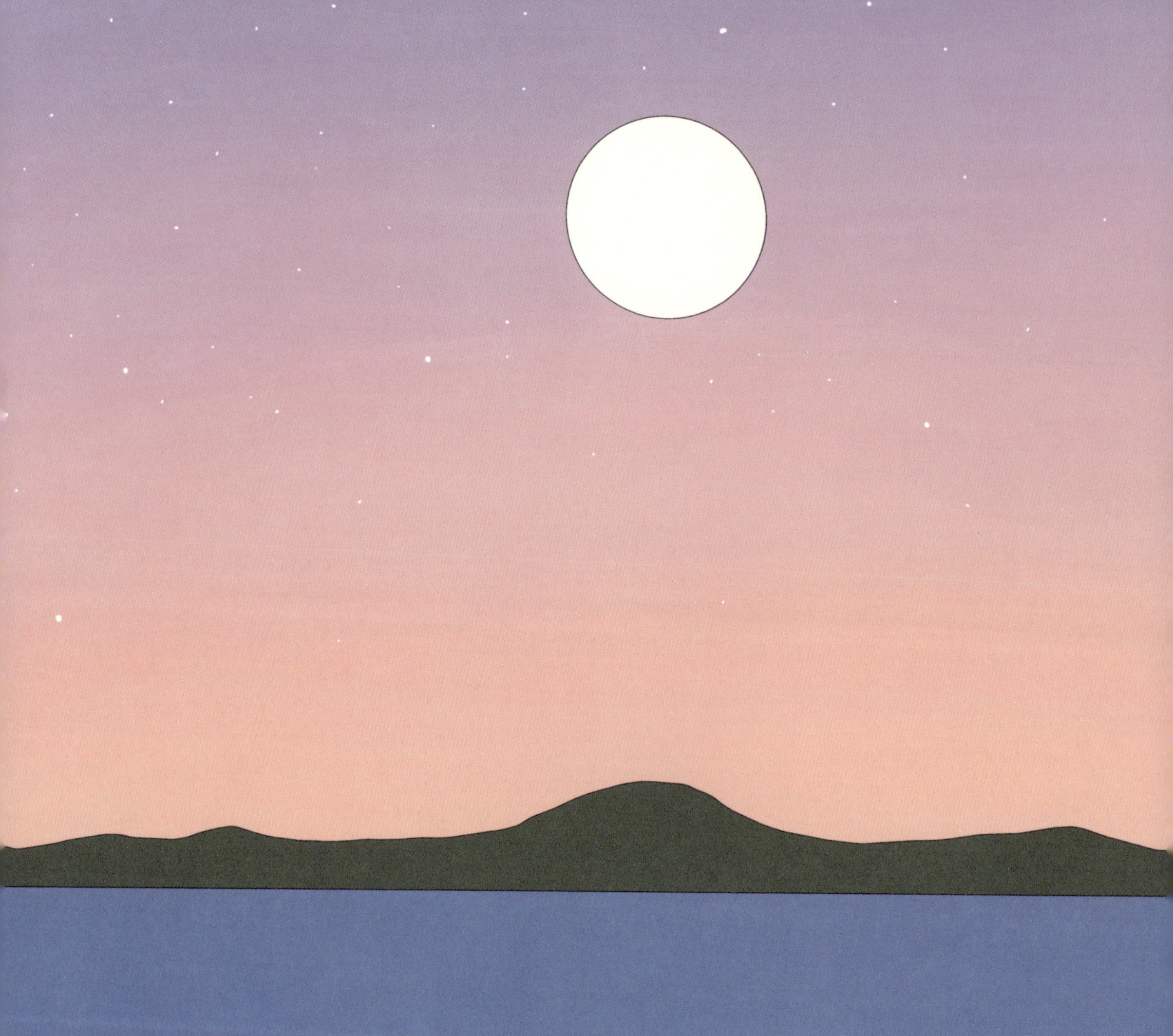

OF SIMPLY BEING IN A BODY.

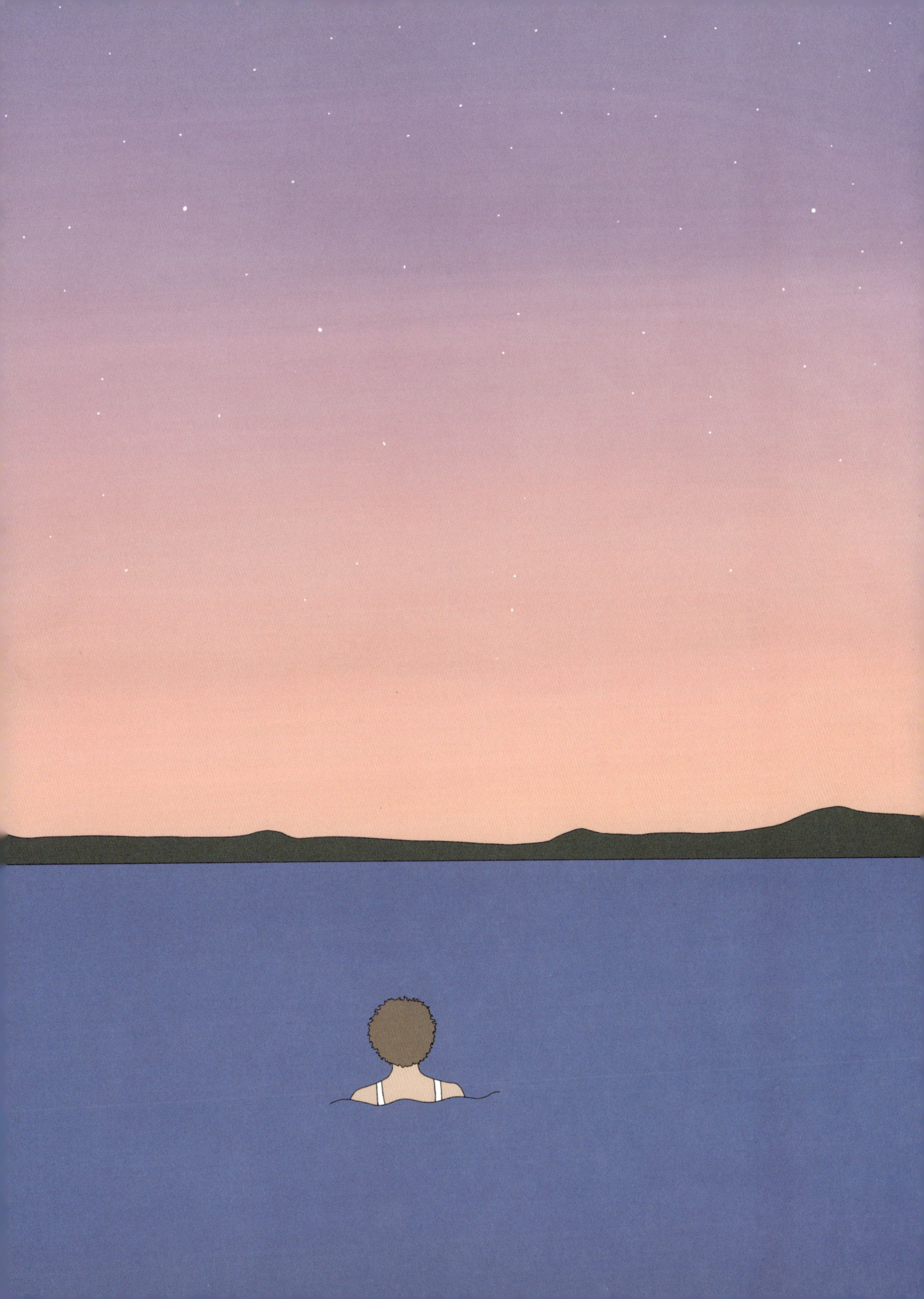

FINDING HELP

1737, NEED TO TALK? — Free call or text. Need to talk? 1737 is free to call or text from any landline or mobile phone, 24 hours a day 7 days a week.

ANXIETY NEW ZEALAND — 0800 ANXIETY (0800 269 4389)

DEPRESSION HELPLINE — 0800 111 757 or free text 4202 (available 24/7)

HEALTHLINE — 0800 611 116

KIDSLINE — 0800 54 37 54 (0800 KIDSLINE) for young people up to 18 years of age (available 24/7)

LIFELINE — 0800 543 354 (0800 LIFELINE) or free text 4357 (HELP) (available 24/7)

PARENT HELP — 0800 568 856 for whānau seeking support, advice and practical strategies on all parenting concerns. Anonymous, non-judgemental and confidential.

RAINBOW YOUTH — (09) 376 4155, available 11am–5pm weekdays.

SUICIDE CRISIS HELPLINE — 0508 828 865 (0508 TAUTOKO) a free, nationwide service available 24/7 that is is operated by highly trained and experienced telephone counsellors who have undergone advanced suicide prevention training.

SUPPORTING FAMILIES IN MENTAL ILLNESS — 0800 732 825

THELOWDOWN.CO.NZ — email team@thelowdown.co.nz or free text 5626

WHAT'S UP — 0800 942 8787 (for 5–18 year olds). Phone counselling is available Monday to Friday, 12 noon–11pm and weekends, 3pm–11pm. Online chat is available from 1pm–10pm Monday to Friday, and 3pm–10pm on weekends.

WWW.DEPRESSION.ORG.NZ — includes The Journal online help service.

YOUTHLINE — 0800 376 633, text 234, talk@youthline.co.nz

ACKNOWLEDGEMENTS

My beautiful mum and dad, thank you for being by my side through it all. Harley, Alice, Joy, Charlotte, Harry, Amelia, Ruby, Samir, Rachel, Luke and Sara, thank you for your endless love and encouragement. Thank you Grace, Cat, Claire and the whole team at Penguin Random House for helping me bring this little book to life. Thank you to every medical worker, school counsellor, carer and teacher working tirelessly to improve the lives of others.

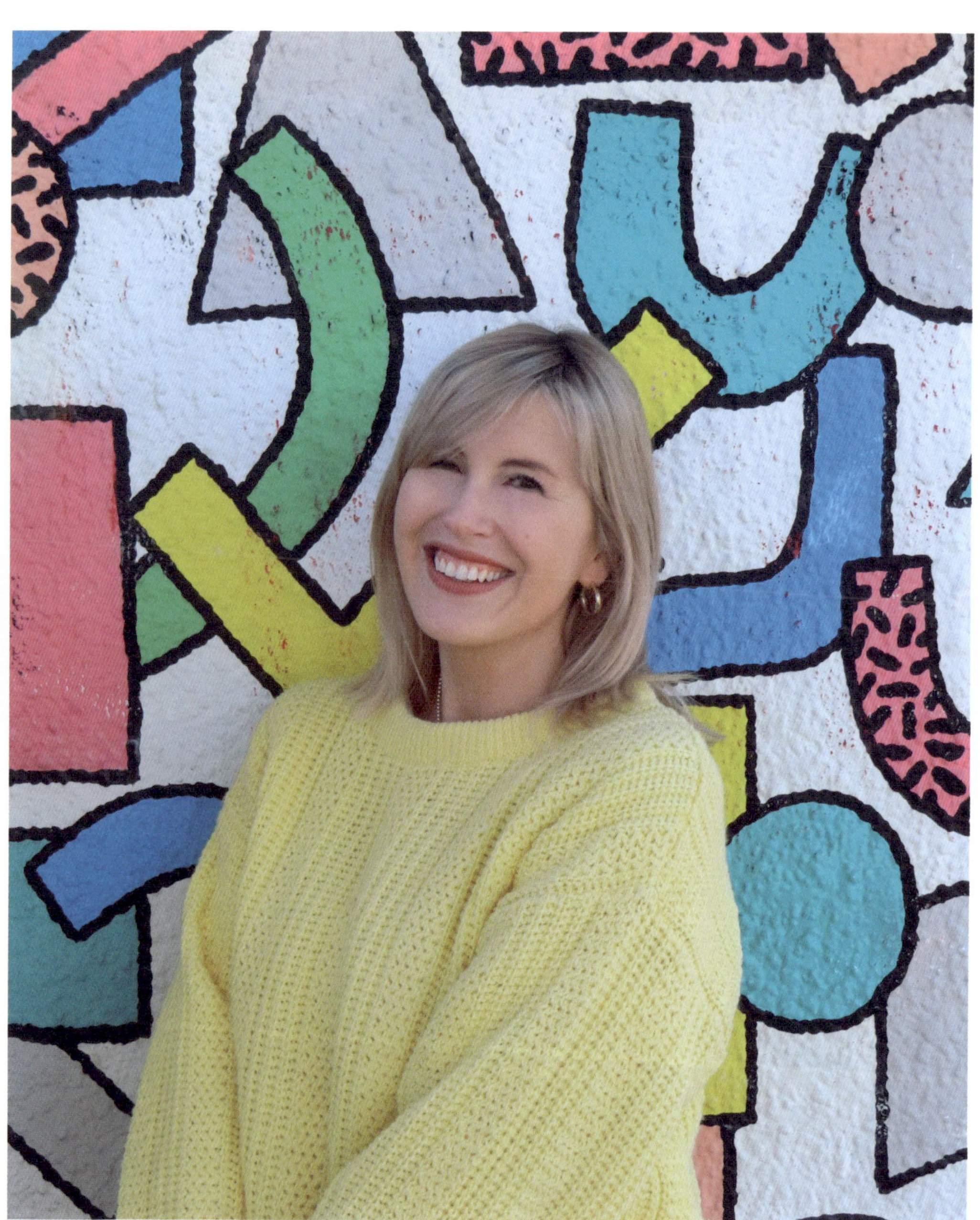

ABOUT THE AUTHOR

Ruby Jones is an illustrator based in Wellington, New Zealand. She likes to make art that shines a little light on everyday moments; our connection to ourselves, each other and the world around us. Ruby is best known for her drawing of two women embracing in a hug with the words 'this is your home and you should have been safe here', which was shared widely following the 2019 Christchurch terror attacks. Following this, Ruby was asked to illustrate a cover for Time magazine and later that same year released her first book and bestseller, All Of This Is For You: A Little Book of Kindness.

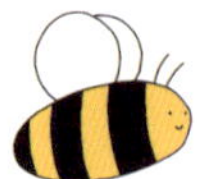

PENGUIN

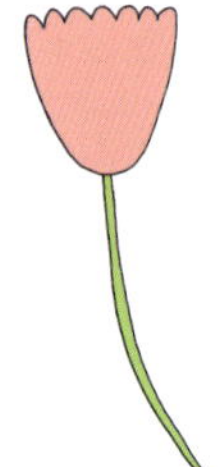

UK | USA | Canada | Ireland | Australia
India | New Zealand | South Africa | China

Penguin is an imprint of the Penguin Random House group of companies, whose addresses can be found at global.penguinrandomhouse.com.

Penguin
Random House
New Zealand

First published by Penguin Random House New Zealand, 2022

1 3 5 7 9 10 8 6 4 2

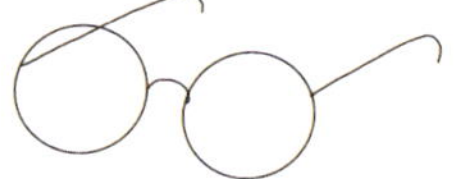

Design by Cat Taylor © Penguin Random House New Zealand
Author photograph by J Moore
Prepress by Soar Communications Group
Printed and bound in China by Toppan Leefung Printing Limited

A catalogue record for this book is available from the National Library of New Zealand.

ISBN 978-1-76104-920-0

penguin.co.nz

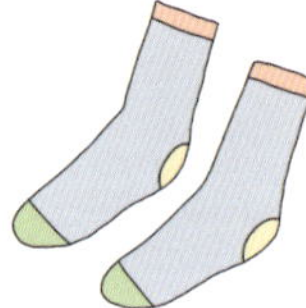

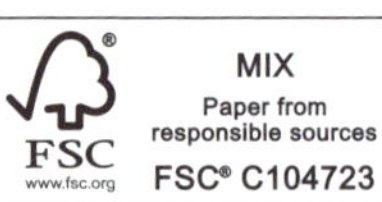

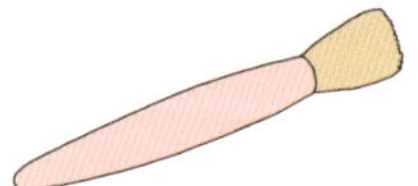

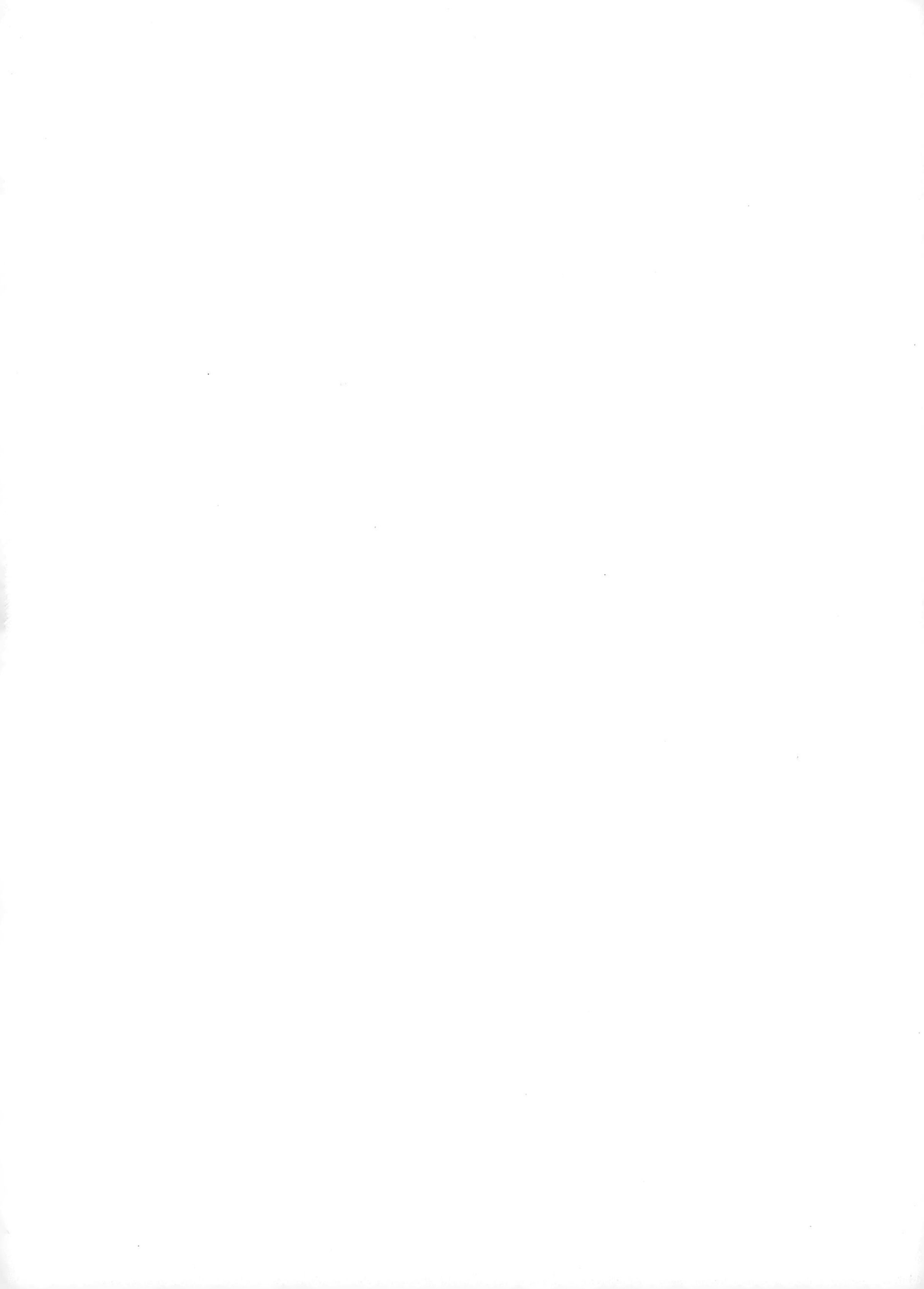